T0227386

INTERVENTIONAL CARDIOLOGY CLINICS

www.interventional.theclinics.com

Editor-in-Chief

MATTHEW J. PRICE

Updates in Percutaneous Coronary Intervention

April 2019 • Volume 8 • Number 2

ELSEVIER

1600 John F. Kennedy Boulevard • Suite 1800 • Philadelphia, Pennsylvania, 19103-2899

http://www.theclinics.com

INTERVENTIONAL CARDIOLOGY CLINICS Volume 8, Number 2
April 2019 ISSN 2211-7458, ISBN-13: 978-0-323-67850-6

Editor: Lauren Boyle
Developmental Editor: Donald Mumford

© **2019 Elsevier Inc. All rights reserved.**

This periodical and the individual contributions contained in it are protected under copyright by Elsevier, and the following terms and conditions apply to their use:

Photocopying
Single photocopies of single articles may be made for personal use as allowed by national copyright laws. Permission of the Publisher and payment of a fee is required for all other photocopying, including multiple or systematic copying, copying for advertising or promotional purposes, resale, and all forms of document delivery. Special rates are available for educational institutions that wish to make photocopies for non-profit educational classroom use. For information on how to seek permission visit www.elsevier.com/permissions or call: (+44) 1865 843830 (UK)/(+1) 215 239 3804 (USA).

Derivative Works
Subscribers may reproduce tables of contents or prepare lists of articles including abstracts for internal circulation within their institutions. Permission of the Publisher is required for resale or distribution outside the institution. Permission of the Publisher is required for all other derivative works, including compilations and translations (please consult www.elsevier.com/permissions).

Electronic Storage or Usage
Permission of the Publisher is required to store or use electronically any material contained in this periodical, including any article or part of an article (please consult www.elsevier.com/permissions). Except as outlined above, no part of this publication may be reproduced, stored in a retrieval system or transmitted in any form or by any means, electronic, mechanical, photocopying, recording or otherwise, without prior written permission of the Publisher.

Notice
No responsibility is assumed by the Publisher for any injury and/or damage to persons or property as a matter of products liability, negligence or otherwise, or from any use or operation of any methods, products, instructions or ideas contained in the material herein. Because of rapid advances in the medical sciences, in particular, independent verification of diagnoses and drug dosages should be made.

Although all advertising material is expected to conform to ethical (medical) standards, inclusion in this publication does not constitute a guarantee or endorsement of the quality or value of such product or of the claims made of it by its manufacturer.

Interventional Cardiology Clinics (ISSN 2211-7458) is published quarterly by Elsevier Inc., 360 Park Avenue South, New York, NY 10010-1710. Months of issue are January, April, July, and October. Subscription prices are USD 203 per year for US individuals, USD 474 for US institutions, USD 100 per year for US students, USD 204 per year for Canadian individuals, USD 565 for Canadian institutions, USD 150 per year for Canadian students, USD 296 per year for international individuals, USD 565 for international institutions, and USD 150 per year for international students. To receive student/resident rate, orders must be accompanied by name of affiliated institution, date of term, and the *signature* of program/residency coordinator on institution letterhead. Orders will be billed at individual rate until proof of status is received. Foreign air speed delivery is included in all *Clinics* subscription prices. All prices are subject to change without notice. **POSTMASTER:** Send address changes to *Interventional Cardiology Clinics*, Elsevier Health Sciences Division, Subscription Customer Service, 3251 Riverport Lane, Maryland Heights, MO 63043. **Customer Service: Telephone: 1-800-654-2452** (U.S. and Canada); **1-314-447-8871** (outside U.S. and Canada). **Fax: 1-314-447-8029. E-mail: journalscustomerservice-usa@elsevier.com (for print support); journalsonlinesupport-usa@elsevier.com (for online support).**

Reprints. For copies of 100 or more of articles in this publication, please contact the Commercial Reprints Department, Elsevier Inc., 360 Park Avenue South, New York, NY 10010-1710. Tel.: 212-633-3874; Fax: 212-633-3820; E-mail: reprints@elsevier.com.

CONTRIBUTORS

EDITOR-IN-CHIEF

MATTHEW J. PRICE, MD
Director, Cardiac Catheterization Laboratory,
Division of Cardiovascular Diseases, Scripps
Clinic, La Jolla, California,
USA

AUTHORS

LAWRENCE ANG, MD
Division of Cardiovascular Medicine, Sulpizio
Cardiovascular Center, University of
California, San Diego, La Jolla,
California, USA

FARNAZ AZARBAL, MD
Division of Cardiovascular Diseases, Scripps
Clinic, La Jolla, California, USA

MATTHEW A. CAVENDER, MD, MPH
Assistant Professor of Medicine, Division of
Interventional Cardiology, The University of
North Carolina at Chapel Hill, Chapel Hill,
North Carolina, USA

RHIAN E. DAVIES, DO
Lifespan Cardiovascular Institute, Rhode
Island Hospital, The Warren Alpert Medical
School of Brown University, Providence,
Rhode Island, USA

MARIO F.L. GAUDINO, MD, FEBCTS
Department of Cardiothoracic Surgery, Weill
Cornell Medicine, NewYork–Presbyterian
Hospital, New York, New York, USA

IAN C. GILCHRIST, MD
Professor of Medicine, Cardiology, Penn State
Heart and Vascular Institute, The Pennsylvania
State University College of Medicine, Hershey,
Pennsylvania, USA

DAVID W. LEE, MD
Interventional Cardiology Fellow, Division of
Interventional Cardiology, The University of
North Carolina at Chapel Hill, Chapel Hill,
North Carolina, USA

MICHAEL S. LEE, MD
UCLA Medical Center, Los Angeles,
California, USA

EHTISHAM MAHMUD, MD
Division of Cardiovascular Medicine,
Sulpizio Cardiovascular Center, University
of California, San Diego, La Jolla, California,
USA

ANTHONY MAIN, MD
Division of Cardiology, Foothills Medical
Centre, University of Calgary, Calgary,
Canada

JAD OMRAN, MD
Division of Cardiovascular Medicine,
Sulpizio Cardiovascular Center, University
of California, San Diego, La Jolla, California,
USA

MITUL PATEL, MD
Division of Cardiovascular Medicine, Sulpizio
Cardiovascular Center, University of
California, San Diego, La Jolla, California, USA

DUANE S. PINTO, MD, MPH
Director of the Cardiac Catheterization
Laboratory, Beth Israel Deaconess Medical
Center, Associate Professor, Harvard Medical
School, Boston, Massachusetts, USA

MATTHEW J. PRICE, MD
Director, Cardiac Catheterization Laboratory,
Division of Cardiovascular Diseases, Scripps
Clinic, Assistant Professor, Scripps
Translational Science Institute, La Jolla,
California, USA

TANVEER RAB, MD, FACC, FSCAI
Professor of Medicine, Interventional
Cardiology, Emory University School of
Medicine, Atlanta, Georgia, USA

RYAN REEVES, MD
Division of Cardiovascular Medicine,
Sulpizio Cardiovascular Center, University
of California, San Diego, La Jolla, California, USA

JACQUELINE SAW, MD, FRCPC, FACC,
FAHA, FSCAI
Interventional Cardiology, Division of
Cardiology, Vancouver General Hospital,
Clinical Professor, University of British Columbia,
Vancouver, British Columbia, Canada

ARNOLD H. SETO, MD, MPA
Department of Medicine, University of
California, Orange, California, USA;
Department of Medicine, Veterans
Administration Long Beach Health Care
System, Long Beach, California, USA

EVAN SHLOFMITZ, DO
MedStar Washington Hospital Center,
Washington, DC, USA

RICHARD SHLOFMITZ, MD
Chairman of Cardiology, St. Francis
Hospital, The Heart Center, Roslyn,
New York, USA

CRISTIANO SPADACCIO, MD, PhD
Department of Cardiothoracic Surgery,
Golden Jubilee National Hospital,
University of Glasgow, Institute of
Cardiovascular and Medical Sciences,
Glasgow, United Kingdom

DAVID P. TAGGART, MD, PhD, FRCS
Department of Cardiovascular Surgery,
University of Oxford, Oxford, United
Kingdom; Department Cardiac Surgery,
John Radcliffe Hospital, Headington,
Oxford, Oxfordshire,
United Kingdom

MARK K. TUTTLE, MD
Interventional Cardiology Fellow, Beth Israel
Deaconess Medical Center, Clinical and
Research Fellow, Harvard Medical School,
Boston, Massachusetts, USA

DANIEL WALTERS, MD
Division of Cardiovascular Medicine,
Sulpizio Cardiovascular Center, University
of California, San Diego, La Jolla, California,
USA

MASOOD YOUNUS, MD
Department of Medicine, University of
California, Orange, California,
USA

CONTENTS

Newer-generation Metallic Stents: Design, Performance Characteristics, and Outcomes

Farnaz Azarbal and Matthew J. Price

Several new coronary stents have been, or soon will be, introduced in the United States. These stents incorporate certain characteristics, such as polymer-free drug coatings, ultrathin stent struts, bioresorbable polymers, and composite materials, that address currently unmet clinical needs to enhance acute stent performance, improve longer-term clinical outcomes, and obviate obligatory prolonged dual antiplatelet therapy. This article reviews the key and novel features of these stents.

Dorsal (Distal) Transradial Access for Coronary Angiography and Intervention

Rhian E. Davies and Ian C. Gilchrist

 Video content accompanies this article at http://www.interventional.theclinics.com.

Access to the arterial system through the distal or dorsal terminal end of the radial artery has recently been developed for interventional and diagnostic procedures. This technique may offer some advantages for specific patient subsets over the traditional radial approach. It may also offer advantages to the operator especially when using the left radial artery. The approach to successful dorsal radial access is described along with hemostasis. Although significant adverse events have not been described in the literature or on social media, several potential areas for vigilance are mentioned.

Clinical Outcomes Data for Instantaneous Wave-Free Ratio-Guided Percutaneous Coronary Intervention

Masood Younus and Arnold H. Seto

Instantaneous wave-free ratio (iFR) is a vasodilator-free index of coronary blood flow used for revascularization decision-making. iFR-based revascularization also had a decreased rate of adverse effects from vasodilators, shorter procedure times, and lower revascularization rates. iFR-pullback predicts post–percutaneous coronary intervention physiologic outcomes in tandem and diffuse coronary lesions. iFR may be particularly useful in patients with potential adenosine resistance, contraindications to adenosine, and multivessel or serial lesions. iFR is a useful tool both with and without fractional-flow reserve for revascularization planning.

Technical Approaches to Left Main Coronary Intervention: Contemporary Best Practices

Tanveer Rab

Left main percutaneous coronary intervention is an acceptable alternative to coronary artery bypass grafting, and in experienced hands, excellent procedural results can be obtained. A systematic approach to stenting and meticulous attention to detail are required. For most lesions, a single-stent provisional approach is sufficient, but for the more complex lesion, a 2-stent technique is required. Herein, the optimal approach to left main lesion assessment and percutaneous intervention is described.

The occupational hazards for interventional cardiologists include the risk of cataracts, malignancy, and orthopedic injury. Robotic technology is now available with the introduction of platforms for performing percutaneous coronary and peripheral interventions. The original remote navigation system has evolved into the current CorPath robotic system, now approved for robotic-assisted cardiovascular interventions. The system removes the operator from the tableside and has been validated for safety, feasibility, and efficacy in coronary and peripheral vascular disease.

Successful percutaneous coronary intervention (PCI) can be challenging in the presence of heavily calcified lesions. Severely calcified lesions are associated with worse clinical outcomes. Recognition of calcification is important before stenting to ensure adequate stent expansion can be attained. Orbital atherectomy is a safe and effective method to ablate calcified plaque. Lesion preparation through plaque modification with orbital atherectomy before stent implantation can help to optimize the results of PCI in these complex lesions.

Despite the progressive expansion of clinical indications for percutaneous coronary intervention and the increasingly high risk profile of referred patients, coronary artery bypass grafting (CABG) remains the mainstay in multivessel disease, providing good long-term outcomes with low complication rates. Multiple arterial grafting, especially if associated with anaortic techniques, might provide the best longer-term outcomes. A surgical approach individualized to the patients' clinical and anatomic characteristics, and surgeon and team experience, are key to excellent outcomes. Current evidence regarding patient selection, indications, graft selection, and potential strategies to optimize outcomes in patients treated with CABG is summarized.

Most patients presenting with myocardial infarction owing to spontaneous coronary artery dissection can be managed conservatively. Revascularization should be pursued in the presence of high-risk features. Percutaneous coronary intervention is preferred over coronary artery bypass grafting, except in left main dissection. Interventionists should exercise extreme caution and meticulous techniques. Using a cutting balloon to fenestrate and decompress the false lumen is appealing and may avoid the need for long stents. Other percutaneous approaches may also be feasible, and interventionists should be familiar with these various approaches when embarking on spontaneous coronary artery dissection percutaneous coronary intervention.

Periprocedural myocardial infarction (MI) occurs infrequently in the current era of percutaneous coronary interventions (PCI) and is associated with an increased risk of mortality and morbidity. Periprocedural MI can occur due to acute side branch occlusion, distal embolization, slow flow or no reflow phenomenon, abrupt vessel closure, and nonidentifiable mechanical processes. Therapeutic strategies to reduce the risk of periprocedural MI include dual antiplatelet therapy, intravenous cangrelor in the periprocedural setting, intravenous glycoprotein IIb/IIIa inhibitor in high-risk patients, anticoagulation with unfractionated heparin, low-molecular-weight heparin or bivalirudin, and embolic protection devices during saphenous vein graft interventions.

ST-elevation myocardial infarction (STEMI) patients with multivessel disease and without shock are a common clinical entity, but the best approach to nonculprit vessel lesions remains controversial. In contrast, STEMI patients with shock do not appear to benefit from primary multivessel percutaneous coronary interventions (PCIs) during the index procedure. The optimal treatment strategy in a given STEMI patient involves an individualized approach, incorporating clinical, hemodynamic, and angiographic/imaging parameters. Patients with STEMI and cardiogenic shock may benefit from therapies other than PCI, such as mechanical cardiovascular support.

UPDATES IN PERCUTANEOUS CORONARY INTERVENTION

RELATED SERIES

Cardiology Clinics
Cardiac Electrophysiology Clinics
Heart Failure Clinics

THE CLINICS ARE NOW AVAILABLE ONLINE!

Access your subscription at:
www.theclinics.com

PREFACE

Percutaneous Coronary Intervention Gathers No Moss

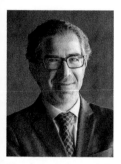

Matthew J. Price, MD
Editor

The identity of the interventional cardiologist has evolved substantially over the past decade, expanding far beyond the realm of angioplasty for the treatment of obstructive coronary atherosclerosis. As I entered our Cardiac Catheterization Laboratory at Scripps Clinic the other day, I was struck by the degree to which our daily practices have changed since I was an interventional fellow at the start of the current century. In one room, an interventional cardiologist and cardiothoracic surgeon were in the midst of performing a transcatheter aortic valve replacement (TAVR); in a second room, another interventional cardiologist was revascularizing the lower extremity of a patient with critical limb ischemia. In a third room, an echocardiographer was performing a transesophageal echocardiogram in a patient with degenerative mitral valve disease who was about to undergo transcatheter mitral valve repair; and in the fourth room, an interventional cardiologist was advancing an Impella catheter into a patient's left ventricle in preparation for a high-risk, complex percutaneous coronary intervention (PCI).

My primary goal as Editor-in-Chief of *Interventional Cardiology Clinics* over the past 3 years has been to provide a comprehensive resource for this modern interventional cardiologist. To that end, the issues have delivered to the reader the current "state-of-the-art" across the diverse range of procedures that we now perform, including but not limited to peripheral vascular intervention, transcatheter mitral valve repair and replacement, TAVR, transcatheter tricuspid valve intervention, and left atrial appendage closure. However, coronary angiography and PCI remain our field's center of gravity despite the excitement that surrounds these new technologies and procedures, encompassing nearly one million procedures per year in the United States alone, driven by device iteration, new adjunctive techniques and pharmacology, and data derived from large-scale randomized clinical trials and observational registries. I admonish my fellows that, as they continue onward in their careers, to never stop learning and to incorporate into their practice new data and ideas, and the current issue of *Interventional Cardiology Clinic* demonstrates that the field of coronary intervention is far from static. I hope, and, indeed, expect, that after reading this "state-of-the-art" of PCI, you will be excited as I am about the present, and future, of coronary angiography and intervention.

Matthew J. Price, MD
Cardiac Catheterization Laboratory
Division of Cardiovascular Diseases
Scripps Clinic
9898 Genesee Avenue
Suite AMP-200
La Jolla, CA 92037, USA

E-mail address:
price.matthew@scrippshealth.org

Intervent Cardiol Clin 8 (2019) ix
https://doi.org/10.1016/j.iccl.2019.01.002
2211-7458/19/© 2019 Published by Elsevier Inc.

Newer-generation Metallic Stents
Design, Performance Characteristics, and Outcomes

Farnaz Azarbal, MD, Matthew J. Price, MD*

KEYWORDS

• Drug-coated stent • Drug-eluting stent • Ridaforolimus • Zotarolimus • Polymer-free stent

---

KEY POINTS

- Despite the excellent outcomes of current drug-eluting stents (DESs), improvements in acute and long-term performance and robust demonstration of the safety of shortened dual antiplatelet therapy (DAPT) in patients at high bleeding risk are desirable goals.
- The BioFreedom polymer-free drug-coated stent, which consists of a 316L stainless steel platform with a microstructured abluminal surface covered with Biolimus A9, was associated with a lower rate of target lesion revascularization and improved safety compared with bare-metal stents in patients at high bleeding risk treated with DAPT, 1 month.
- The Osiro DES is an ultrathin L-605 cobalt chromium stent with a biodegradable polymer that elutes sirolimus; in a large, randomized trial, this stent was noninferior, and possibly superior, for target lesion failure compared with the Xience durable-polymer everolimus-eluting stent, driven by reductions in periprocedural myocardial infarction.
- The EluNir DES consists of an L-605 cobalt chromium platform with variable strut thickness and adaptive cells that elutes ridaforolimus from a polyurethane/poly n-butyl methacrylate polymer blend; a large randomized clinical trial demonstrated that the EluNir DES was noninferior to Resolute Integrity zotarolimus-eluting stent (ZES) for the endpoints of angiographic late luminal loss (LLL) and target vessel failure.
- The Resolute Onyx ZES is an iteration of Resolute ZES, consisting of a composite wire of cobalt chromium and a dense inner core of platinum iridium, with thinner stent struts that have a swaged shape; in a prospective study, LLL was noninferior and superior to a historical Resolute ZES control.
- The Resolute Onyx 2.0-mm stent was associated with a low rate of target lesion failure and in-stent LLL consistent with that of prior-generation ZESs in lesions with larger reference vessel diameter, without a signal for stent thrombosis.

INTRODUCTION

Since the advent of intracoronary stent placement for the treatment of obstructive coronary artery disease (CAD), many technological advances have been made to improve acute performance and long-term patient outcomes. Drug-eluting stents (DESs) were developed to reduce the rate of coronary restenosis seen with bare-metal stents (BMSs). Despite the excellent outcomes with current-generation DESs, several limitations remain. Although DESs reduce restenosis, they are also associated with chronic vascular inflammation and stent thrombosis (ST), a phenomenon that underpins the rationale for prolonged

---

Division of Cardiovascular Diseases, Scripps Clinic, 9898 Genesee Avenue, AMP-200, La Jolla, CA 92037, USA
* Corresponding author.
E-mail address: price.matthew@scrippshealth.org

Intervent Cardiol Clin 8 (2019) 95–109
https://doi.org/10.1016/j.iccl.2018.11.001
2211-7458/19/© 2018 Elsevier Inc. All rights reserved.

postprocedure dual antiplatelet therapy (DAPT) with aspirin and an oral platelet P2Y$_{12}$ receptor antagonist. This requirement is a particular problem in patients at high risk of bleeding or in those who require urgent surgery. Despite the indirect evidence of improved safety with the latest generation of DESs, robust prospective data are lacking supporting very short DAPT (ie, 1 month) in this patient population. Furthermore, as more complex coronary anatomy is tackled in the cardiac catheterization laboratory, improved acute performance, radial strength, deliverability, fluoroscopic visualization, and ability to treat extremes in coronary artery size remain important goals in the development of new stent technology.

The aims of this review are to describe the important and novel features of 4 new-generation metallic stents: BioFreedom (Biosensors International, Morges, Switzerland), Orsiro (Biotronik, AG, Bülach, Switzerland), EluNIR (Medinol, Tel Aviv, Israel), and Resolute Onyx (Medtronic, Santa Rosa, California) (Table 1). For each stent type, the platform, antiproliferative drug, and polymers used are described and key studies pertaining to clinical safety and efficacy highlighted.

BIOFREEDOM POLYMER-FREE DRUG-COATED STENT

DESs control the delivery of antiproliferative drug to the intima over a specific time course and concentration using polymer elution kinetics. DESs with durable polymers (DPs) are associated with persistent fibrin deposition, greater inflammation, and poorer endothelialization, resulting in delayed arterial healing compared with BMSs.[1] Both DPs and biodegradable polymers (BPs) have been associated with local arterial hypersensitivity reactions that may contribute to late thrombosis.[2,3] The presence of a drug-carrying polymer necessitates prolonged use of DAPT to prevent ST, limiting DES use in individuals at elevated risk of bleeding. The BioFreedom stent is drug-coated stent (DCS) that delivers its antiproliferative agent without the use of a polymer. The goal of a polymer-free (PF) DCS is to provide the same inhibition of neotiminal hyperplasia via controlled, localized antiproliferative drug delivery as a DES without the adverse consequences of a drug-carrying polymer.

Platform

The BioFreedom PF-DCS stent uses a 316L, polished stainless steel BioFlex II stent platform with a stent strut thickness of 112 μm. The abluminal side is modified to create a microstructured surface that permits the drug to adhere to the stent without the use of a polymer (Fig. 1). The drug is coated specifically on the vessel wall side to minimize release into the lumen and impairment of endothelialization. Study of release kinetics demonstrates 90% drug release from the stent within 48 hours of implantation, with the remaining drug released within 28 days.[4,5] After the drug is completely absorbed by the vessel wall, a BMS remains.

Antiproliferative Drug

The characteristics of the antiproliferative agent used in DCS are critical given the rapid release from the PF microstructured stent surface compared with the slower elution kinetics seen with DESs. Umirolimus, also known as Biolimus A9 (BA9), is the antiproliferative drug used in the BioFreedom PF-DCS. It is a semisynthetic, 31-membered triene macrolide lactone derivative of sirolimus. It inhibits cell growth through inhibition of the mammalian target of rapamycin (mTOR), which is a protein kinase that controls cell growth, proliferation, and survival. Sirolimus analogs form a complex with cytoplasmic proteins that in turn inhibit the cell cycle between the G0 and G1 phases to interrupt cell growth and proliferation. BA9 is a highly liphophilic drug, permitting easy crossing of the cell membrane. This lipophilicity is critical to maintained sustained concentrations within the intimal wall after its rapid release from the metal scaffold. Consistent with this, the tissue concentration of BA9 in porcine arteries at 28 days after implantation of BioFreedom PF-DCS is comparable to that of DP-DESs.[5] Moreover, there is low systemic exposure to BA9 compared to the Cypher sirolimus-eluting stent (SES).[6]

Preclinical Data

Tada and colleagues[4] performed a preclinical study to assess the ability of BioFreedom PF-DCS stents to inhibit neointimal proliferation and to quantify the vascular inflammation associated with the stent in a porcine overstretch coronary model. They compared high-dose (HD) (225-μg/14-mm BA9) and low-dose (LD) (112-μg/14-mm BA9) PF-DCS with both the Cypher DP SES (Cordis Corporation) and a BMS. A pathologist blinded to treatment arms measured neointimal thickness and tabulated a vessel injury score by quantifying the fibrin deposition, granulomas, and giant cells around the stent struts. Two of 17 animals had detectable serum BA9 levels at 28 days; at 180 days, all animals had

Table 1
Newer-generation metallic stent characteristics

Stent Name	Platform Material	Strut Size (μm)	Coating Thickness (μm)	Polymer	Drug	Special Features
BioFreedom	316L SS	112	10	None	BA9 (15.6 μg/mm)	Drug-coated, no drug-eluting polymer
Osiro	CoCr	60	7.4	PLLA	Sirolimus (1.4 μg/mm^2)	BP, thinnest struts
EluNir	CoCr	87	7	Poly n-butyl methacrylate	Ridaforolimus (1.1 μg/mm^2)	
Onyx	CoCr shell, platinum iridium core	81	6	C10 polymer, C19 polymer, and polyvinyl pyrrolidinone	Zotarolimus (1.6 μg/mm^2)	Composite core improves radiopacity; available in 2.0-mm diameter size

Abbreviations: CoCr, cobalt-chromium; SS, stainless steel.

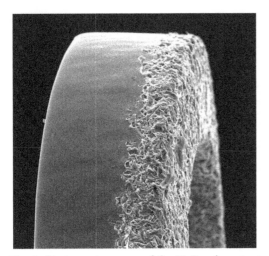

Fig. 1. Electron microscopy of the BioFreedom stent platform with microstructured abluminal surface. (*Adapted from* Tada N, Virmani R, Grant G, et al. Polymer-free BA9-coated stent demonstrates more sustained intimal inhibition, improved healing, and reduced inflammation compared with a polymer-coated sirolimus-eluting cypher stent in a porcine model. Circ Cardiovasc Interv 2010;3(2):175; with permission.)

serum BA9 concentrations below the lower limit of quantitation. At 180 days, 0.02% of the original BA9 dose remained on the BioFreedom stents (Fig. 2). Compared with the SES, both doses of BioFreedom stents were associated with reduced neointimal proliferation (neointimal thickness: HD, 0.12 mm $\pm$ 0.034 mm; LD, 0.10 mm $\pm$ 0.040 mm; SES, 0.20 mm $\pm$ 0.111 mm; BMS, 0.17 mm $\pm$ 0.099 mm; P<.001) and were associated with significantly decreased fibrin deposition and local inflammation.

Clinical Studies

Costa and colleagues[5] published the first-in-human (FIH) evaluation in a prospective, randomized study of the performance, safety, and efficacy of the BioFreedom PF-DCS compared with the first-generation Taxus Liberté paclitaxel-eluting stent (PES, Boston Scientific). The study examined 2 different doses of BA9: standard dose (SD) (15.6 μm/mm of stent length) and LD (7.8 μg/mm of stent length). A total of 182 patients with stable ischemic symptoms or a positive functional study were randomized to treatment with PF-DCS SD, PF-DCS LD, or PES. The primary endpoint was in-stent late luminal loss (LLL) at 12-month angiographic follow-up. The PF-DCS SD group, but not the PF-DCS LD group, demonstrated noninferiority versus PES for LLL (PF-DCS SD 0.17 mm vs PES 0.35 mm; P<.001). At 5 years there were no significant

differences in major adverse cardiovascular events (MACEs) or clinically indicated target lesion revascularization (TLR) across the 3 group and no episodes of Academic Research Consortium (ARC)-defined definite/probable ST, although the study was not powered to detect noninferiority or differences in clinical endpoints. The BioFreedom FIM trial, therefore, supports the safety and antirestenotic efficacy of the PF-DCS stent in stable coronary disease, although it is a small study of patients with simple coronary lesions. The SD stent was further studied in trials powered to assess clinical outcomes.

The Prospective Randomized Comparison of the BioFreedom Biolimus A9 Drug-Coated Stent Versus the Gazelle Bare-Metal Stent in Patients at High Bleeding Risk (LEADERS FREE) trial was a randomized, double-blind, multicenter study that comprises the largest clinical study of the BioFreedom PF-DCS stent to date.[7] The study recruited patients with a clinical indication for percutaneous coronary intervention (PCI), including acute coronary syndrome (ACS), and who were considered to be at high bleeding risk (HBR) with prolonged DAPT. HBR was based on several criteria, such as advanced age (>75 years), concurrent anticoagulation, recent hemorrhage, chronic anemia, chronic kidney disease, and cancer. A total of 2466 patients were enrolled and randomized to receive either PF-DCS or a BMS (Gazelle, Biosensors Interventional, Morges, Switzerland). Patients received 1-month DAPT post-PCI. The primary safety endpoint was a composite of cardiac death, myocardial infarction (MI), and ST. The primary efficacy endpoint was clinically driven TLR. At 390-day follow-up, the PF-DCS was superior to BMS for the primary safety endpoint (9.4% vs 12.9%; P = .005), primarily driven by a lower rate of MI in the PF-DCS group (both periprocedural and spontaneous). The PF-DCS patients also experienced significantly lower rates of clinically driven TLR (5.1% vs 9.8%; P<.001). The treatment effect of the PF-DCS for both safety and efficacy was consistent across most subgroups. There was a particular benefit in safety with PF-DCS in the ACS subgroup (P interaction = 0.04), and a particular benefit in efficacy with PF-DCS in patients with renal failure (P interaction = 0.02). The LEADERS FREE findings support the efficacy of the BioFreedom PF-DCS over BMS and the safety of a very short course of DAPT after PF-DCS implantation in HBR patients. Among study participants, 64% percent were considered at HBR solely on the basis of advanced age. In contemporary practice, such patients may not uniformly be considered at

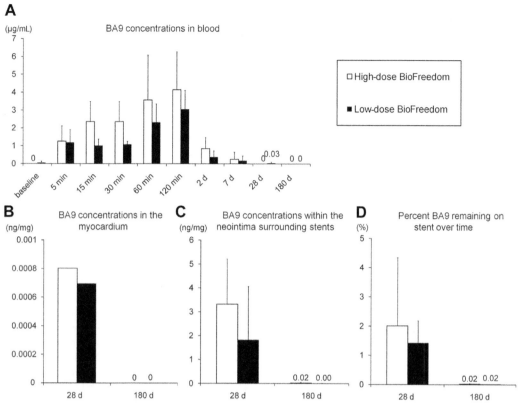

Fig. 2. BA9 concentration in blood (*A*), myocardium (*B*), neointima surrounding stents (*C*), and stents (*D*) over time in both HD (225-µg/14-mm) and LD (112-µg/14-mm) BioFreedom PF drug-coated stents. The HD is used in the commercially available BioFreedom stent. (*Adapted from* Tada N, Virmani R, Grant G, et al. Polymer-free Biolimus A9-coated stent demonstrates more sustained intimal inhibition, improved healing, and reduced inflammation compared with a polymer-coated sirolimus-eluting cypher stent in a porcine model. Circ Cardiovasc Interv 2010;3(2):177; with permission.)

prohibitive risk for use of a current DESs, particularly given increasing evidence of safety with shorter durations of DAPT. However, robust data to support 1-month DAPT after current DESs are currently lacking. The 2-year outcomes of LEADERS FREE demonstrated sustained safety and efficacy benefits of PF-DCS over BMS.[8]

Use with anticoagulation

The performance of the BioFreedom PF-DCS in individuals on concurrent long-term oral anticoagulation (OAC) was explored in a LEADERS FREE substudy.[9] A total of 879 (35.6%) of the trial participants were scheduled to remain on OAC after PCI. In this subgroup, the PF-DCS was associated with a lower rate of 2-year TLR compared with BMS (7.9% vs 11.2%; *P* = .0514), whereas there were no significant differences in safety (14.4% vs 15.0%; *P* = not significant [NS]) or in the rate of major bleeding (10.7% vs 12.9%; *P* = NS). The generalizability of

these findings is limited by the increasing use of non–vitamin K OACs (NOACs), because more than 91% of patients were treated with warfarin, although clinical trials have demonstrated a significantly increased risk of bleeding in patients treated with NOACs and single-antiplatelet or dual-antiplatelet therapy. Furthermore, most OAC-treated patients in LEADERS FREE received triple therapy with aspirin, clopidogrel, and warfarin for the first 30-days post-PCI, whereas only 6.6% of participants were treated with dual therapy of clopidogrel and warfarin without aspirin, as per the What is the Optimal Antiplatelet and Anticoagulant Therapy in Patients with Oral Anticoagulation and Coronary Stenting (WOEST) trial. A North American consensus document recommends post-PCI treatment with triple therapy (OAC or NOAC and DAPT) for 1 month or more in patients with balanced thrombotic and bleeding risk or high thrombotic and low bleeding risk, whereas OAC (or NOAC) and 1 antiplatelet agent immediately after PCI in patients at HBR and low thrombotic risk.[10]

Polymer-free DCS in acute coronary syndrome

The outcomes of BioFreedom PF-DCS in patients with ACS have been reported in 2 studies. In a prespecified substudy of the 659 ACS patients enrolled in the LEADERS FREE trial,[11] 12-month TLR was significantly reduced with PF-DCS compared with BMS (3.9% vs 9.0%; P = .009). The PF-DCS arm also demonstrated superior safety, with a lower rate of cardiac death, MI, or definite/probable ST (9.3% vs 18.5%; P = .001), driven by lower rates of cardiac mortality (3.4 vs 6.9%; P = .049) and MI (6.9 vs 13.8%; P = .005). The 2-year outcomes of this population were reported by Jensen and colleagues.[12] Between the first and second years of follow-up, there was no significant difference in the occurrence of the safety endpoint between groups (PF-DCS, 11 patients, vs BMS, 8 patients; P = .560). Similarly, between year 1 and year 2 there was no significant difference in the occurrence of the efficacy endpoint between groups (PF-DCS, 3 patients, vs BMS, 4 patients; P = .152). Based on these results, the investigators concluded that with the availability of PF-DCS, the use of BMS in HBR patients presenting with ACS can no longer be recommended.

The Biolimus-Eluting Stent in Patients with ST-Segment Elevation Acute Myocardial Infarction in Metropolitan Public Hospital (BESAMI MUCHO) study was a single-center, observational study that enrolled 175 consecutive patients presenting with ST elevation MI (STEMI) treated with the BioFreedom PF-DCS followed by 12-month DAPT.[13] The investigators propose that use of a PF-DCS in the context of an STEMI is of particular clinical interest because the emergent context may preclude thorough assessment of the relative contraindications to long-term DAPT, leading to potential risk in the case of premature discontinuation. At 1-year follow-up, the rate of cardiac death, recurrent MI, and ischemia-driven target vessel revascularization was 4.6%. In-hospital ST occurred in 2 patients. Of the 70 patients who underwent 6-month angiographic follow-up, the average LLL was 0.13 mm ± 0.14 mm, comparable to contemporary DESs.[14,15] DAPT interruption occurred in 10% of the enrolled patients before 1 year, without adverse clinical consequence.

All-comer populations

Safety and Efficacy of Polymer-Free Biolimus-Eluting Stents in All-Comer Patients: the RUDI-FREE Study[16] was a prospective, observational, multicenter study conducted in Italy that enrolled 1104 patients undergoing PCI with the PF-DCS stent. Approximately 60% of the enrolled population presented with stable CAD, 27% with non-ST elevation ACS, and 13% with STEMI. HBR was present in 16.3%. DAPT was recommended for 12 months post-PCI in the majority of patients (55%). At 1-year follow-up, the primary endpoint (a composite of cardiovascular death, MI, and definite/probable ST) occurred in 4.1% of patients, definite/probable ST occurred in 1.1%, and TLR occurred in only 1.2%. The findings of this large registry further support the safety and efficacy of PF-DCS in a non-HBR cohort predominantly treated with longer-duration DAPT.

Future Directions

Although published studies support the safety and efficacy of the BioFreedom PF-DCS stent followed by 1-month DAPT in stable CAD as well as ACS, important clinical questions remain. Several studies seek to confirm the findings of the LEADERS FREE trial. SORT OUT IX is a randomized multicenter trial that will compare the safety and efficacy of BioFreedom PF-DCS with that of the Osiro BP-SES in approximately 3150 patients with stable CAD or ACS (NCT02623140). The objectives of the prospective, multicenter, open-label, single-arm LEADERS FREE II trial are to confirm the safety of the PF-DCS with 1-month DAPT followed by aspirin alone and to confirm superiority with respect to TLR compared with BMS (NCT02843633). The trial will enroll approximately 1200 HBR patients in North America and Europe. The control arm of the study is the BMS group of the LEADERS FREE trial, and outcomes will be compared using propensity-score adjustment. The results of the LEADERS FREE II study will be used to seek Food and Drug Administration (FDA) approval for the commercial use of the BioFreedom PF-DCS in the United States.

Other considerations regarding the data for the PF-DCS include the observation that the struts of the comparator BMS in the LEADERS FREE trial are relatively thick (112 μm), which may have contributed to relative efficacy of the PF-DCS. In addition, it is unknown how PF-DCS or other PF stents may perform in comparison to second-generation DP-DESs, because prior studies have only compared PF-DCS to DP-SES,[6] DP-PES,[5] and BMS.[7–9,11,12,17] The safety of 1-month DAPT after second-generation DES has not been robustly and prospectively evaluated in a large clinical trial, however. The Randomized Controlled Trial With Resolute Onyx in One Month Dual Antiplatelet Therapy for High-Bleeding Risk Patients (ONYX ONE) will randomize approximately 2000 HBR patients undergoing PCI to either the Onyx DES or the Bio-Freedom PF-DCS; both arms will receive 1-month DAPT. The primary endpoint is a composite of cardiac death, MI, and definite/probable ST at 1 year, and the powered secondary endpoint is target lesion failure (TLF) at 1 year (NCT03344653). Other ongoing trials of 1-month DAPT after newer DESs in HBR patients include XIENCE 28 (NCT03355742). The EVOLVE Short DAPT Study is a prospective, multicenter, single-arm study designed to assess the safety of 3-month DAPT in HBR subjects undergoing PCI with the Synergy (Boston Scientific) BP-EES.

ORSIRO BIODEGRADABLE POLYMER DRUG-ELUTING STENT

The Orsiro stent was recently approved by the FDA for use in the United States. Similar to the BioFreedom PF-DCS, Orsiro stent technology attempts to mitigate vascular inflammation induced by chronic exposure to a drug-eluting polymer. Rather than removing the polymer from the stent surface, however, Orsiro uses a BP to preserve the mechanism of drug elution without long-term polymer exposure.

Platform
The Orsiro stent platform consists of an ultrathin L-605 cobalt chromium alloy PRO-Kinetic Energy stent. The stent is composed of helical struts, with adjacent loops connected by 3 longitudinal struts. The uncoated stent struts are 60-μm thick, which are the thinnest of the currently available metallic stents. The polymer-coated struts for stents less than or equal to 3.0 mm in diameter are 71-μm thick, and the struts of stents greater than 3.0 mm in diameter are 91-μm thick.[18] Such thin struts may improve stent flexibility, integration with the vessel wall, re-endothelialization, reduced peristrut inflammation and injury, ST, and restenosis.[19–21]

Antiproliferative Drug
The Osiro BP-DES stent elutes sirolimus (rapamycin), a cytostatic agent that binds to FK binding protein 12 (FKBP-12); this complex then binds to and inhibits the activation of mTOR, which, by inhibiting cell-cycle progression from the G1 to the S phase, reduces vascular smooth muscle cell proliferation and in turn reduces neointimal hyperplasia. The antirestenotic efficacy of sirolimus was well demonstrated by the Cypher DP-SES.

Biodegradable Polymer
The bare-metal scaffold of the Osiro stent is coated with 2 distinct components (**Fig. 3**). The outer layer is poly-L-lactic acid (PLLA) BP that delivers sirolimus at a concentration of $1.4 \ \mu g/mm^2$. The PLLA-sirolimus matrix is coated 7.5-μm thick on the abluminal surface and 3.5-μm thick on the luminal surface of the scaffold. The drug is released over 3 months after implantation, with 50% released during the first 30 days.[22] Within 24 months, the PLLA polymer degrades into carbon dioxide and water, leaving behind the second component of the stent coating, a passive coating of silicon carbide that encapsulates the stent. The silicon carbide is intended to act as a diffusion barrier to seal the bare-metal surface and minimize its interaction with the endothelial surface, minimizing metal ion release and thus accelerating re-endothelialization.[23,24]

Clinical Studies
Early studies
The Biotronik-Safety and Clinical Performance of the Drug Eluting Orsiro Stent in the Treatment of Subjects With Single De Novo Coronary Artery Lesions (BIOFLOW)-I study was an FIH exploratory assessment of the Orsiro BP-SES stent in 30 subjects.[18] The study was conducted at 2 centers in Romania and enrolled patients

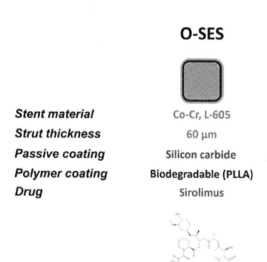

O-SES	
Stent material	Co-Cr, L-605
Strut thickness	60 μm
Passive coating	Silicon carbide
Polymer coating	Biodegradable (PLLA)
Drug	Sirolimus

Fig. 3. Composition of Orsiro stent platform. Co-Cr, cobalt-chromium; O-SES, Orsiro sirolimus-eluting stent. (*Adapted from* Windecker S, Haude M, Neumann FJ, et al. Comparison of a novel biodegradable polymer sirolimus-eluting stent with a durable polymer everolimus-eluting stent: results of the randomized BIOFLOW-II trial. Circ Cardiovasc Interv 2015;8(2):e001441; with permission.)

with unstable angina, stable angina, or silent ischemia who had a single de novo lesion in 1 coronary artery. Mean in-stent LLL at 9-month follow-up angiography, the primary endpoint of the study, was only 0.05 mm ± 22 mm. Clinically driven TLR occurred in 2 (6.7%) of 30 participants, noted to be outside the stent but within the stented segment (ie, within 5 mm of a stent edge). MACEs at 1 year occurred in 10%, including 1 cardiac death and 2 cases of ischemia-driven TLR. No MIs or STs were observed.

The BIOFLOW-II trial was a multicenter, randomized, noninferiority study that randomly assigned 452 patients undergoing PCI to the Orsiro BP-SES or the DP Xience everolimus-eluting stent (EES) in a 2:1 fashion.[22] The BP-SES was found noninferior to the DP-EES for the primary endpoint LLL at 9 months (0.10 mm ± 0.32 mm vs 0.11 mm ± 0.29 mm; P noninferiority <0.0001). In the prespecified cohorts undergoing intravascular imaging (optical coherence tomography [n = 65] or intravascular ultrasound [n = 66]) neointimal thickness, neointimal area, and the proportion of uncovered or malapposed struts were similar between groups. There were no significant differences between BP-SES and the DP-EES in the rates of TLF (6.5% vs 8.0%; P = .58), cardiac death (0.7% vs 0.7%; P = .98), target-vessel MI (2.7% vs 2.6%; P = .95), or TLR (3.5% vs 4.7%; P = .54). There were no cases of ST in either group.

Observational studies
Several studies have evaluated the efficacy of the Orsiro BP-SES in complex lesions and in ACS. BIOFLOW-III was a prospective, observational, multicenter registry of 1356 high-risk patients undergoing PCI with the BP-SES, including those with acute MI, chronic total occlusions, left main stenosis, and multivessel disease.[25] The primary endpoint of TLF (a composite of cardiac death, target vessel MI, coronary artery bypass graft surgery, and clinically driven TLR) at 12 months occurred in 5.1% of the participants, compared with 10.0% in BIOFLOW-I and 6.5% in BIOFLOW-II. The rate of definite ST was 0.2%.

Clinical outcomes with BP-SES in a broader range of patients was explored in the Comparison of Biodegradable Polymer and Durable Polymer Drug-eluting Stents in an All Comers Population: Randomized Multicenter Trial in an All Comers Population Treated Within the Netherlands (BIO-RESORT), which was a 3-arm, randomized, noninferiority study of Orsiro BP-SES compared with the Resolute DP

zotarolimus-eluting stent (ZES) and the Synergy BP-EES. The study enrolled 3514 all-comer patients at 4 clinical sites in the Netherlands. Approximately 70% of participants presented with ACS; 31% presented with STEMI. The primary endpoint was a composite of cardiac death, target vessel MI, or target vessel revascularization at 12 months. At 12-month follow-up, the rate of the primary endpoint was 5% in all 3 groups. Both of the BP stents met the criteria for noninferiority compared with the Resolute Integrity DP-EES (both absolute risk difference −0.7%; 95% CI, −2.4–1.1; upper limit of 1-sided 95% CI, 0.8%; P noninferiority <0.0001). ARC-defined definite ST occurred in 0.3% of each stent group.

Randomized trials powered for clinical outcomes
The clinical efficacy of the Osiro BP-SES compared with contemporary DESs was first examined in the Sirolimus-eluting Stents With Biodegradable Polymer vs an Everolimus-eluting Stents (BIOSCIENCE) noninferiority trial, which randomly assigned 2119 patients undergoing PCI for stable CAD or ACS to either BP-SES or Xience DP-EES.[26] At 12-month follow-up, the primary endpoint (TLF) was noninferior with BP-SES compared with Xience DP-EES (6.5% vs 6.6%; P noninferiority <0.0004), and the rates of ST were not significantly different (0.9% vs 0.4%). There was a significant treatment interaction in the prespecified subgroup of patients presenting with STEMI, in whom there seemed particular benefit with BP-SES (rate of TLF, 3.3% vs 8.7%; P = .024; P interaction = 0.014). At 2-year follow-up, the observed benefit of BP-SES in the STEMI cohort was sustained, with a lower risk of TLF (5.4% vs 10.8%), driven mainly by numerically lower rates of cardiac death or MI.[27]

BIOFLOW V was a large, international, randomized, bayesian noninferiority trial designed in consultation with the FDA with the intention of generating sufficient data for Orsiro approval in the United States.[28] The trial randomized 1334 patients in 2:1 fashion to undergo percutaneous revascularization with the Orsiro BP-SES or Xience DP-EES. The primary endpoint was TLF, defined as a composite of cardiovascular death, target vessel–related MI, or ischemia-driven TLR. The statistical analysis combined data from these patients and those from BIOFLOW II (N = 452) and BIOFLOW IV (N = 579) to achieve adequate statistical power and used a noninferiority margin of 3.85%. At 12-month follow-up, the rate of TLF with BP-SES was both noninferior and superior to DP-EES (6% vs 10%, posterior probability for noninferiority 100%, and post hoc posterior probability for superiority 96.5%) (Fig. 4).

Although the results of BIOFLOW V strongly support the safety and efficacy of Orsiro BP-SES compared with contemporary DP-DES technology, there are several limitations. The lower incidence of the primary endpoint in the Orsiro group was driven by lower rates of periprocedural MI, as defined by elevated levels of cardiac enzymes. The clinical significance of these silent periprocedural infarctions is unclear. Furthermore, procedural characteristics between the 2 groups differed, because the DP-EES group had significantly greater length of implanted stents, total number of implanted stents, and prevalence of overlapping stents—all predictors of periprocedural MI that were not accounted for by the randomization process. Adjusted analyses accounting for these procedural differences, however, were consistent with the overall findings of the trial, with lower rates of TLF and target lesion MI with the BP-SES, and there was no observed treatment interaction according to lesion characteristics. Another potential limitation is the higher-than-previously observed rate of TLF in the DP-EES group, a chance finding that may have favored BP-SES.

Future Directions

There are several ongoing clinical trials comparing head-to-head outcomes of Orsiro BP-SES with other contemporary DESs. For example, the Bioresorbable Polymer ORSIRO vs Durable Polymer RESOLUTE ONYX Stents (BIONYX) trial (NCT02508714) is a prospective, randomized, noninferiority, single-blind, multicenter trial randomizing 2470 all-comer patients to PCI with Orsiro BP-SES or Resolute Onyx DP-ZES.

ELUNIR DRUG-ELUTING STENT

Platform

The metal platform of the EluNIR DES is composed of L-605 cobalt chromium with struts 87 μm in thickness. The strut width is variable, with both wide (72-μm) and narrow (40-μm) struts depending on the cell location (Fig. 5). This variability in strut width is intended to confer device flexibility while maintaining radial strength. The adaptive cells of the platform are capable of differential lengthening to provide uniform drug distribution in variable vessel anatomy.

Antiproliferative Drug

The antiproliferative drug used in the EluNIR stent is the rapamycin-derivative ridaforolimus, which forms a complex with the cytoplasmic protein FKBP-12, which in turn inhibits mTOR. Ridaforolimus seems to have superior in vitro antiproliferative effects on vascular smooth muscle cells with relative preservation of vascular endothelial cell function when compared with zotarolimus, sirolimus, and everolimus.[29] The drug concentration is 1.1 μm/mm^2 of stent.

Polymer

The drug-eluting polymer used by the EluNIR DES is a 55%/45% blend of thermoplastic

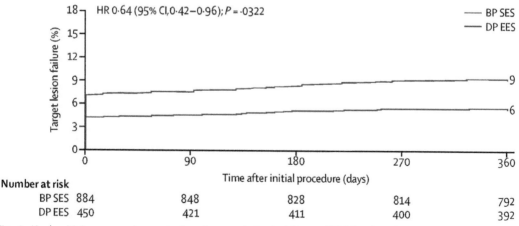

Fig. 4. Kaplan-Meier curves demonstrating the cumulative incidence of TLF for the BP-SES versus DP-EES in the BIOFLOW V randomized clinical trial. (*Reprinted with permission from* Elsevier (The Lancet, Kandzari DE, Mauri L, Koolen JJ, et al. Ultrathin, bioresorbable polymer sirolimus-eluting stents versus thin, durable polymer everolimus-eluting stents in patients undergoing coronary revascularisation [BIOFLOW V]: a randomised trial. Lancet 2017;390(10105):1849.)

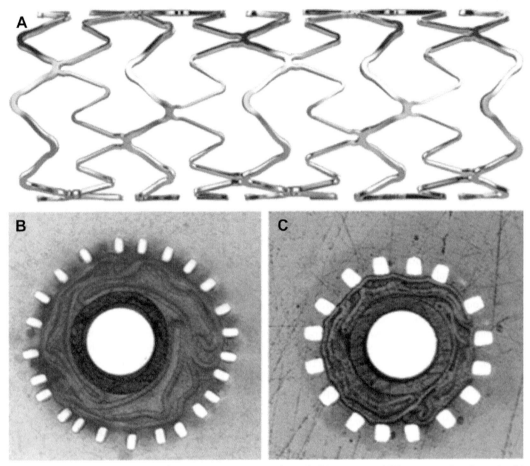

Fig. 5. EluNIR DES. (A) Longitudinal view, (B) cross-section through thin struts, and (C) cross-section through wide struts. (*Adapted from* Paradies V, Ben-Yehuda O, Jonas M, et al. A prospective randomized trial comparing the novel ridaforolimus-eluting BioNIR stent to the zotarolimus-eluting Resolute stent: 6 months angiographic and 1 year clinical results of the NIREUS trial. EuroIntervention 2018;14(1):87; with permission.)

silicone polycarbonate polyurethane and poly n-butyl methacrylate. The latter is also a component of the Cypher SES; it demonstrates elastomeric properties that are intended to minimize disruptions in polymer integrity during stent expansion. The thickness of the copolymer coating is 7 μm. Rather than an initial burst of drug release, ridaforolimus is eluted at a relatively more gradual and steady rate over time. Approximately half the drug content is released by 14 days postimplant, and 98% of the drug is eluted over 180 days (Fig. 6).

Clinical Studies

The outcomes of the FIH results of the BioNIR stent were reported in the Angiography Study of BioNIR Drug Eluting Stent System (NIREUS) trial.[30] This study was a prospective, randomized, single-blind, multicenter noninferiority trial involving 31 centers in Europe and Israel. Patients undergoing PCI were randomly assigned in a 2:1 fashion to receive either the BioNIR ridaforolimus-eluting stent (RES) or the Resolute Integrity ZES. The primary endpoint was in-stent LLL at 6-month angiography. A total of 302 patients were enrolled, with 85% undergoing angiographic follow-up. In-stent LLL at 6 months was similar between groups (BioNIR RES, 0.04 mm ± 0.31 mm, vs Resolute ZES, 0.03 mm ± 0.31 mm; noninferiority $P<.0001$). There were no significant differences between groups in death, TLF, TVF, or MACEs at 1-year follow-up. There was 1 case of ST in the BioNIR RES group, attributed to DAPT noncompliance.

The BioNIR Ridaforolimus-Eluting Coronary Stent System in Coronary Stenosis (BIONICS) trial was a prospective, randomized, single-blind, multicenter noninferiority trial powered to assess the clinical outcomes of BioNIR RES compared with Resolute ZES to seek device approval by the FDA. The study enrolled a total of 1919 patients, including those with complex

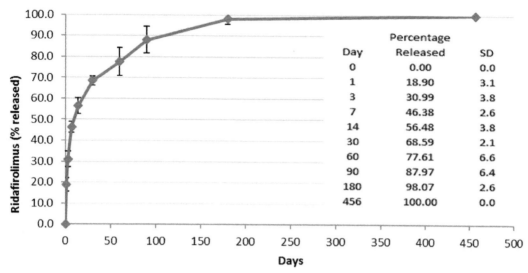

Day	Percentage Released	SD
0	0.00	0.0
1	18.90	3.1
3	30.99	3.8
7	46.38	2.6
14	56.48	3.8
30	68.59	2.1
60	77.61	6.6
90	87.97	6.4
180	98.07	2.6
456	100.00	0.0

Fig. 6. Release kinetics of ridaforolimus from the EluNIR DES in an in vivo porcine model. Slightly more than half of the ridaforolimus content is released by 14 days postimplant, approximately 90% is released by 90 days (87.97%), and approximately all is released by 180 days. (*Adapted from* Kandzari DE, Smits PC, Love MP, et al. Randomized comparison of ridaforolimus- and zotarolimus-eluting coronary stents in patients with coronary artery disease: primary results from the BIONICS Trial (BioNIR Ridaforolimus-Eluting Coronary Stent System in Coronary Stenosis). Circulation 2017;136(14):1304–14; with permission.)

coronary lesions, such as calcific lesions requiring atherectomy, bypass graft stenosis, chronic total occlusions, and BMS restenosis. The primary endpoint was TLF, defined as the composite of cardiac death, target vessel MI, or ischemia-driven TLR. Secondary endpoints included MACEs, TVF, and individual components of the composite endpoints. The trial was powered for an estimated TLF rate of 5.8% and a noninferiority margin of 3.3%. At 12-month follow-up, the rate of the primary endpoint was 5.4% in both stent groups (P noninferiority = 0.001). There were no significant differences in the rates of the individual components of the composite clinical outcomes. Among the 158 patients enrolled in the angiographic substudy, 13-month LLL was similar between groups (BioNIR RES 0.22 mm ± 0.41 mm vs Resolute ZES 0.23 mm ± 0.41 mm; P noninferiority = 0.004). In the intravascular ultrasound substudy of 111 patients, there was no significant difference in percent of neointimal hyperplasia (BioNIR RES 8.1% ± 5.8% vs Resolute ZES 8.9% ± 7.8%; P noninferiority = 0.01). Given these results, the EluNir RES was subsequently approved by the FDA for commercial use in the United States.

RESOLUTE ONYX DRUG-ELUTING STENT

Platform

The Resolute Onyx DES is an iteration of the Resolute DES family. A single, continuous strand of wire material with a composite core with a swaged shape is formed into a sinusoidal design, helically wrapped around a mandrel and laser fused at specific crowns to form the final stent scaffold. The wire material is a composite of a platinum iridium core with a cobalt alloy shell. The highly dense inner core, composed of 90% platinum and 10% iridium, enhances stent visibility despite a reduction in strut thickness compared with prior iterations (Fig. 7). The strut thickness is 81 μm for the 2.25-mm to 4.0-mm diameter sizes. Compared with the predecessor, Resolute Integrity, the Onyx DES features thinner struts but with a larger strut width-to-thickness ratio to maintain radial strength. The objectives of these changes to the metal backbone are to improve acute and long-term performance by decreasing strut thickness while maintaining radiopacity and radial strength, thereby reducing neointimal hyperplasia and geographic miss. The Onyx stent is uniquely available in smaller (2.0-mm) and larger (4.5-mm and 5.0-mm) diameter sizes.

Antiproliferative Drug and Durable Polymer

The Onyx stent elutes the lipophilic mTOR inhibitor zotarolimus from the BioLinx (Medtronic) DP. BioLinx is a blend of 3 different polymers: the hydrophobic C10 polymer, which aids in the control of drug release; the hydrophilic C19 polymer, which supports biocompatibility; and polyvinyl pyrolidinone, which increases initial drug burst

A

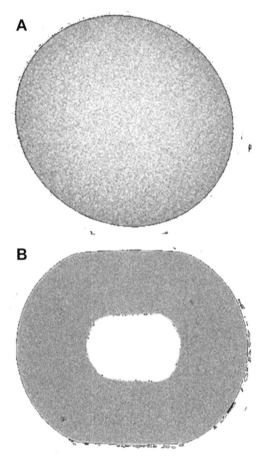

B

Fig. 7. Cross-sectional strut of the Resolute Integrity and Resolute Onyx. (A) Resolute Integrity; (B) Resolute Onyx. Cobalt alloy shown in gray and platinum-iridium shown in white. Note the swaged shape of the Onyx strut. Images are not to scale. (*Adapted from* Price MJ, Saito S, Shlofmitz RA, et al. First report of the resolute Onyx 2.0-mm zotarolimus-eluting stent for the treatment of coronary lesions with very small reference vessel diameter. JACC Cardiovasc Interv 2017;10(14):1383; with permission.)

and enhances the elution rate.[31] Compared with Resolute Integrity, Onyx uses the same delivery polymer, antiproliferative drug, and dose density. Due to geometric changes in the scaffold, however, it delivers a slightly reduced overall drug load at most stent sizes. In porcine models of the prior iteration of the Resolute stent, the polymer elutes 85% of the zotarolimus content during the first 60 days after implantation, with the remaining drug eluted within the first 180 days.

Clinical Data

The RESOLUTE ONYX core study explored the angiographic effectiveness of the Onyx ZES.[32] The study was a prospective, single-arm, noninferiority trial performed at 12 centers in the United States, using propensity-adjusted results of the angiographic cohort of the RESOLUTE US clinical trial as a historical control. The study enrolled 75 patients with stable or unstable angina or a positive stress test and up to 2 target lesions in separate vessels. Patients with ACS or requiring staged PCI were excluded. Enrolled patients underwent repeat angiography at 8 months. The primary endpoint was in-stent LLL. Secondary endpoints included clinical outcomes, such as cardiac death, target vessel MI, TLR, and ST. In-stent LLL at 8 months was both noninferior and significantly lower with Onyx ZES compared with the historical Resolute control (0.24 mm ± 0.39 mm vs 0.36 mm ± 0.52 mm; P for superiority = 0.029). Among the lesions enrolled in the intravascular ultrasound substudy, incomplete stent apposition at 8-month follow-up was present in 2 of 20 lesions (10%), both of which were present acutely and at follow-up (ie, persistent incomplete stent apposition), and neointimal hyperplastic percent volume obstruction was 6.88% ± 8.00%. At 8-month follow-up, the rate of TLF was 6.7% and of TLR 4%. Target vessel MI occurred in 2 patients (2.7%) both of which were periprocedural MIs. ST occurred in 1 patient on the day of the index procedure. Subsequent to these findings, the FDA approved the Onyx ZES for commercial use in the United States.

Price and colleagues[33] described the safety and efficacy outcomes of the Onyx 2.0-mm ZES, which, at the time of the study, was a smaller diameter than any DES commercially available in the United States. Outcomes with this stent size are of particular clinical interest because of the known strong association between reference vessel diameter, restenosis, and TLF after PCI. The RESOLUTE ONYX 2.0 Clinical Study was a single-arm, open-label, multicenter study conducted at clinical sites within the United States and Japan. A total of 101 subjects with evidence of ischemic heart disease and up to 2 target lesions amenable to treatment with a 2.0-mm stent were enrolled. The target lesion required a reference vessel diameter greater than or equal to 2.0 mm and less than 2.25 mm by visual estimate. For patients with multivessel disease, a positive functional study involving the area subtended by the target lesion (eg, fractional flow reserve measurement) was required for the subject to be enrolled. Individuals with ACS or planned staged PCI were excluded. Participants underwent clinical follow-up at 12 months and angiographic follow-up was performed in a subset at

13 months. The primary endpoint was TLF at 12-month follow-up, defined as a composite of TLR, target vessel MI, and cardiac death. The mean reference vessel diameter of the enrolled lesions was only 1.91 mm ± 0.26 mm, and 47% of the enrolled patients were diabetic, consistent with a complex lesion and patient cohort. At 12 months, the rate of TLF was 5.0%, the rate of TLR was 2.0%, and the rate of target vessel MI was 3.0%. Despite the small reference vessel diameter of the lesions enrolled, there were no incidences of ST. In the subgroup of patients who underwent follow-up angiography at 13 months, in-stent LLL was 0.26 mm ± 0.48 mm. Rates of restenosis were comparable to reports of the prior-generation Resolute DES implanted in vessels with larger reference diameters. Despite the excellent in-stent LLL with the Onyx 2.0-mm ZES, in-segment percent diameter stenosis and the rate of in-stent binary restenosis were relatively high (37.92% ± 21.54% and 12%, respectively). This may reflect the presence of diffuse disease around target lesions located in the distal coronary tree and the absence of headroom for even small amounts of late loss when implanting a stent within a vessel of such narrow caliber. Although this did not seem to have a clinical impact on 1-year outcomes, a greater duration of follow-up is required to determine whether progression of inflow and/or outflow disease, or continued in-stent late loss, may influence longer-term outcomes.

Outcomes of the Onyx ZES in the setting of ACS were described by Kim and colleagues.[34] The aim of this retrospective, multicenter, observational Korean study was to compare clinical outcomes with Onyx ZES to the Xience EES in the setting of acute MI. A total of 1486 patients who had undergone successful PCI were enrolled: 402 treated with Onyx ZES and 1084 treated with Xience EES. The primary endpoint was TLF, defined as a composite of TLR, target lesion MI, or cardiac death. At 6-month clinical follow-up, there was no significant difference in the adjusted risk for TLF between stents (4.0% vs 3.9%, adjusted hazard ratio [HR] 1.36; 95% CI, 0.67–2.77; P = .930). Rates of the individual components of the composite endpoint as well as ST were also similar between groups.

SUMMARY

Despite excellent outcomes with current DESs, several limitations remain. The new-generation metallic stents feature technologic advances intended to improve acute and long-term performance through changes in the metal backbone and by overcoming vascular injury and the chronic vascular inflammation associated with contemporary DESs. The BioFreedom PF BA9-coated stent seems safer and reduces TLR compared with BMS in patients at high bleeding risk treated with only 1 month of DAPT postimplantation. TLF with the Osiro DES, an ultrathin, BP-SES, was noninferior to, and by post hoc analysis, superior to the gold-standard Xience DP-EES, although the latter finding requires further confirmation. The EluNIR DES, a DP-RES, seems noninferior to DP-EES, thereby providing greater competition in the marketplace. The Onyx ZES, an iteration of the Resolute ZES, incorporates changes to the metal scaffold that may improve acute performance, and a 2.0-mm size demonstrated acceptable clinical outcomes in the treatment of vessels with very small reference diameters, thereby expanding the armamentarium of the interventional cardiologist to treat a challenging lesion subset.

REFERENCES

1. Joner M, Finn AV, Farb A, et al. Pathology of drug-eluting stents in humans: delayed healing and late thrombotic risk. J Am Coll Cardiol 2006;48(1): 193–202.
2. Virmani R, Guagliumi G, Farb A, et al. Localized hypersensitivity and late coronary thrombosis secondary to a sirolimus-eluting stent: should we be cautious? Circulation 2004;109(6):701–5.
3. van der Giessen WJ, Lincoff AM, Schwartz RS, et al. Marked inflammatory sequelae to implantation of biodegradable and nonbiodegradable polymers in porcine coronary arteries. Circulation 1996; 94(7):1690–7.
4. Tada N, Virmani R, Grant G, et al. Polymer-free biolimus a9-coated stent demonstrates more sustained intimal inhibition, improved healing, and reduced inflammation compared with a polymer-coated sirolimus-eluting cypher stent in a porcine model. Circ Cardiovasc Interv 2010;3(2):174–83.
5. Costa RA, Abizaid A, Mehran R, et al. Polymer-free biolimus A9-coated stents in the treatment of de novo coronary lesions: 4- and 12-month angiographic follow-up and final 5-year clinical outcomes of the prospective, multicenter biofreedom FIM clinical trial. JACC Cardiovasc Interv 2016;9(1):51–64.
6. Ostojic M, Sagic D, Jung R, et al. The pharmacokinetics of Biolimus A9 after elution from the Nobori stent in patients with coronary artery disease: the NOBORI PK study. Catheter Cardiovasc Interv 2008;72(7):901–8.
7. Urban P, Meredith IT, Abizaid A, et al. Polymer-free drug-coated coronary stents in patients at high bleeding risk. N Engl J Med 2015;373(21):2038–47.

8. Garot P, Morice MC, Tresukosol D, et al. 2-year outcomes of high bleeding risk patients after polymer-free drug-coated stents. J Am Coll Cardiol 2017;69(2):162–71.

9. Carrié D, Menown I, Oldroyd K, et al. Safety and efficacy of polymer-free biolimus A9-coated versus bare-metal stents in orally anticoagulated patients: 2-year results of the LEADERS FREE oral anticoagulation substudy. JACC Cardiovasc Interv 2017; 10(16):1633–42.

10. Angiolillo DJ, Goodman SG, Bhatt DL, et al. Antithrombotic therapy in patients with atrial fibrillation undergoing percutaneous coronary intervention: a North American perspective-2016 update. Circ Cardiovasc Interv 2016;9(11) [pii:e004395].

11. Naber CK, Urban P, Ong PJ, et al. Biolimus-A9 polymer-free coated stent in high bleeding risk patients with acute coronary syndrome: a Leaders Free ACS sub-study. Eur Heart J 2017;38(13):961–9.

12. Jensen CJ, Naber CK, Urban P, et al. 2-year outcomes of high bleeding risk patients with acute coronary syndrome after biolimus-A9 polymer-free drug-coated stents: a leaders free sub-study. EuroIntervention 2018;13(16):1946–9.

13. Sgueglia GA, D'Errico F, Gioffrè G, et al. Angiographic and clinical performance of polymer-free biolimus-eluting stent in patients with ST-segment elevation acute myocardial infarction in a metropolitan public hospital: the BESAMI MUCHO study. Catheter Cardiovasc Interv 2018;91(5):851–8.

14. Meredith IT, Worthley S, Whitbourn R, et al. Clinical and angiographic results with the next-generation resolute stent system: a prospective, multicenter, first-in-human trial. JACC Cardiovasc Interv 2009; 2(10):977–85.

15. Serruys PW, Ong AT, Piek JJ, et al. A randomized comparison of a durable polymer Everolimus-eluting stent with a bare metal coronary stent: the SPIRIT first trial. EuroIntervention 2005;1(1): 58–65.

16. Sardella G, Stefanini GC, Briquori C, et al. Safety and efficacy of polymer-free biolimus-eluting stents in all-comer patients: the RUDI-FREE study. EuroIntervention 2018;14(7):772–9.

17. Filipovic-Pierucci A, Durand-Zaleski I, Butel T, et al. Polymer-free drug-coated coronary stents are cost-effective in patients at high bleeding risk: economic evaluation of the LEADERS FREE trial. EuroIntervention 2018;13(14):1688–95.

18. Hamon M, Niculescu R, Deleanu D, et al. Clinical and angiographic experience with a third-generation drug-eluting Orsiro stent in the treatment of single de novo coronary artery lesions (BIOFLOW-I): a prospective, first-in-man study. EuroIntervention 2013;8(9):1006–11.

19. Kastrati A, Mehilli J, Dirschinger J, et al. Intracoronary stenting and angiographic results: strut thickness effect on restenosis outcome (ISAR-STEREO) trial. Circulation 2001;103(23):2816–21.

20. Pache J, Kastrati A, Mehilli J, et al. Intracoronary stenting and angiographic results: strut thickness effect on restenosis outcome (ISAR-STEREO-2) trial. J Am Coll Cardiol 2003;41(8):1283–8.

21. Guagliumi G, Musumeci G, Sirbu V, et al. Optical coherence tomography assessment of in vivo vascular response after implantation of overlapping bare-metal and drug-eluting stents. JACC Cardiovasc Interv 2010;3(5):531–9.

22. Windecker S, Haude M, Neumann FJ, et al. Comparison of a novel biodegradable polymer sirolimus-eluting stent with a durable polymer everolimus-eluting stent: results of the randomized BIOFLOW-II trial. Circ Cardiovasc Interv 2015;8(2): e001441.

23. Dahm JB, Willems T, Wolpers HG, et al. Clinical investigation into the observation that silicon carbide coating on cobalt chromium stents leads to early differentiating functional endothelial layer, increased safety and DES-like recurrent stenosis rates: results of the PRO-Heal Registry (PRO-Kinetic enhancing rapid in-stent endothelialisation). EuroIntervention 2009;4(4):502–8.

24. Kalnins U, Erglis A, Dinne I, et al. Clinical outcomes of silicon carbide coated stents in patients with coronary artery disease. Med Sci Monit 2002; 8(2):PI16–20.

25. Waltenberger J, Brachmann J, van der Heyden J, et al. Real-world experience with a novel biodegradable polymer sirolimus-eluting stent: twelve-month results of the BIOFLOW-III registry. EuroIntervention 2016;11(10):1106–10.

26. Pilgrim T, Heg D, Roffi M, et al. Ultrathin strut biodegradable polymer sirolimus-eluting stent versus durable polymer everolimus-eluting stent for percutaneous coronary revascularisation (BIOSCIENCE): a randomised, single-blind, non-inferiority trial. Lancet 2014;384(9960):2111–22.

27. Piccolo R, Heg D, Franzone A, et al. Biodegradable-polymer sirolimus-eluting stents versus durable-polymer everolimus-eluting stents in patients with acute ST-segment elevation myocardial infarction: insights from the 2-year follow-up of the BIOSCIENCE trial. JACC Cardiovasc Interv 2016;9(9):981–3.

28. Kandzari DE, Mauri L, Koolen JJ, et al. Ultrathin, bioresorbable polymer sirolimus-eluting stents versus thin, durable polymer everolimus-eluting stents in patients undergoing coronary revascularisation (BIOFLOW V): a randomised trial. Lancet 2017;390(10105):1843–52.

29. Kandzari DE, Smits PC, Love MP, et al. Randomized comparison of ridaforolimus- and zotarolimus-eluting coronary stents in patients with coronary artery disease: primary results from the BIONICS trial

(BioNIR Ridaforolimus-Eluting Coronary Stent System in Coronary Stenosis). Circulation 2017; 136(14):1304–14.

30. Paradies V, Ben-Yehuda O, Jonas M, et al. A prospective randomized trial comparing the novel ridaforolimus-eluting BioNIR stent to the zotarolimus-eluting resolute stent: six-month angiographic and one-year clinical results of the NIREUS trial. EuroIntervention 2018;14(1):86–93.

31. Udipi K, Chen M, Cheng P, et al. Development of a novel biocompatible polymer system for extended drug release in a next-generation drug-eluting stent. J Biomed Mater Res A 2008;85(4):1064–71.

32. Price MJ, Shlofmitz RA, Spriggs DJ, et al. Safety and efficacy of the next generation Resolute Onyx zotarolimus-eluting stent: primary outcome of the RESOLUTE ONYX core trial. Catheter Cardiovasc Interv 2018;92(2):253–9.

33. Price MJ, Saito S, Shlofmitz RA, et al. First report of the resolute Onyx 2.0-mm Zotarolimus-eluting stent for the treatment of coronary lesions with very small reference vessel diameter. JACC Cardiovasc Interv 2017;10(14):1381–8.

34. Kim Y, Oh SS, Jeong MH, et al. Comparison of short-term clinical outcomes between Resolute Onyx zotarolimus-eluting stents and everolimus-eluting stent in patients with acute myocardial infarction: results from the Korea Acute Myocardial infarction Registry (KAMIR). Cardiol J 2018. https://doi.org/10.5603/CJ.a2018.0053.

Dorsal (Distal) Transradial Access for Coronary Angiography and Intervention

Rhian E. Davies, DO[a], Ian C. Gilchrist, MD[b],*

KEYWORDS

• Dorsal radial artery • Distal radial artery • Snuffbox • Vascular access • Radial access
• Vascular intervention

KEY POINTS

• The distal radial artery sweeps behind the base of the thumb to the anatomic snuffbox, where it is known as the dorsal radial artery.
• The dorsal radial artery is about 80% of the diameter of that found in the forearm and for many patients is large enough to be used as a vascular access site.
• Optimal positioning of the hand for dorsal radial access places the patient in a more natural and relaxed arm position than standard radial access, offering greater comfort.
• Ergonomics for left radial access are better by the dorsal approach compared with traditional radial access.
• Dorsal access is a very new technique that holds promise, but its risks are as yet not well defined.

 Video content accompanies this article at http://www.interventional.theclinics.com.

INTRODUCTION

During the early years of interventional cardiology, the femoral artery held sway as the access site of choice with few other options. Advancements in sheath technology, guide catheter designs, and the interventionalists' desire to provide patients with quicker recovery time and a more pleasant catheterization experience fostered migration to the transradial approach. In comparison studies, patients repeatedly report that a cardiac catheterization via the transradial approach leads to better quality of life after the procedure and overall increased satisfaction with their hospital experience compared with the transfemoral approach. Further driving the shift from femoral to radial access has been the repeated demonstration that transradial access can not only reduce hospital costs but also result in superior outcomes when compared with femoral access.

Radial artery access has many advantages but also has its challenges. Most radial access is obtained from the right radial artery based on tradition and logistical setup of the catheterization laboratory. However, what if the right radial access is not available? Perhaps it is occluded from a prior procedure, has been incorporated into a dialysis fistula, or maybe the patient has an orthopedic condition that prevents appropriate positioning for comfortable sheath placement in the right wrist.[1] For these patients, the left radial artery is a viable alternative to avoid the legacy femoral approach.

Left radial artery access has always had some supporters even in the early transradial

---

R.E. Davies has intellectual property rights to the DRAWS (Davies Precision Machining, Lebanon, PA) arm support device discussed in article and noted in the article.
[a] Lifespan Cardiovascular Institute, Rhode Island Hospital, Warren Alpert Medical School of Brown University, 593 Eddy St, Providence, RI 02903, USA; [b] Cardiology, Penn State Heart and Vascular Institute, The Pennsylvania State University College of Medicine, C1517, 500 University Drive, Hershey, PA 17033, USA
* Corresponding author.
E-mail address: lcg1@psu.edu

2211-7458/19/© 2018 Elsevier Inc. All rights reserved.

development because this access was thought to be more femoral-like than the right radial approach. It is beneficial and even preferred in certain situations, such as when patients are known to have previously undergone coronary artery bypass grafting, in particular, those who had their left internal mammary artery used as a graft to their native left system.[2] The use of the left radial artery also has its challenges, especially in regards to patient and physician comfort. A patient's body habitus may be a limiting factor with overall success much greater when excess abdominal adipose tissue is not present. With left-sided access, patients are often asked to have their arm propped in an uncomfortable position and supinated at the shoulder and elbow for the interventionalist to work with the radial artery. Poorly positioned patient arms can affect the stance of the operator and result in an uncomfortable posture and threaten back injury. As operators and their assistants need to reach over the patient without lying down on top of them, the occupational strain on the lower back can become problematic.

One technique to mitigate some of these challenges has been the realization that the distal radial artery, otherwise known as the dorsal radial artery, within the anatomic snuffbox can be a viable access site to the arterial system. Using this location to access the radial artery obviates wrist supination and results in increased comfort for both the patient and the staff. The advantages and challenges of this approach are the subjects of this article.

HISTORY

The concept that the dorsal radial might be useful for clinical care surfaced in the late 1970s as an alternative access site for arterial monitoring in pediatric patients.[3] Subsequently, there were a variety of case reports and small series primarily in the anesthesia and critical care literature.[4–9] Use of the dorsal radial for cardiovascular imaging and intervention first started in Russia[10] and Iran and subsequently surfaced on Twitter posts. Reports by Kiemeneij[11] and Davies and Gilchrist[1] appeared in peer-review format online in 2017 followed by others[12–15] as a widespread discussion continued through 2017 to 2018 on Twitter and other social media, highlighting a much broader experience. It is this rapid dissemination by Twitter of the dorsal radial approach that is perhaps most notable because it eclipsed the traditional meeting and publication formats that new ideas have typically spread among cardiologists.

ANATOMY

The radial artery originates in most people within the antecubital fossa and runs down the radial side of the forearm until it reaches the wrist near the base of the thumb (Fig. 1A). From here, the main vessel does not continue into the palm but takes a course around the back side of the base of the thumb, eventually passing between the metacarpal bones of the thumb and first finger into the palmar arches (Fig. 1B). The dorsal radial artery is palpable within the junction of the intersection of the thumb and first finger over the bony structures of the snuffbox between tendon bands that control the hand muscles (Fig. 2). At this location on the dorsal aspect of the wrist, the average arterial diameter is 80% of that of the artery in the classical wrist entry site, with a mean diameter of 2.5 mm (range 1.5–4.1 mm) by ultrasound.[16] This range of arterial diameters would suggest that although some may not have dorsal arteries large enough to use, most will have adequate dorsal radial diameters to allow standard diagnostic and interventional work. Beyond the inherently smaller size of this more distal arterial branch, the dorsal radial access site is also

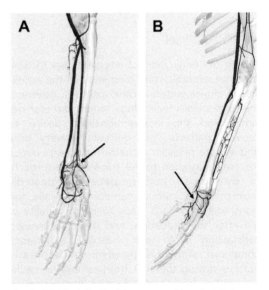

Fig. 1. (A) The left distal forearm and hand with the extremity slightly rotated from the palm up position. The arrow points to junction where the dorsal radial starts to pass behind the base of the thumb, whereas a palmar branch continues into the palmar arch system. (B) The left distal forearm as viewed from the radial side of the forearm. The arrow points to the dorsal radial passing between the first and second metacarpal bones in the anatomic snuffbox, eventually passing up to the palmar arches. Branches are seen feeding wrist bones.

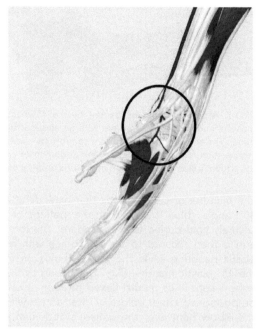

Fig. 2. The tendon and arterial vascular structures at the region of the snuffbox. This is circled in black.

several centimeters further from the central circulation, which may be a potential problem if the equipment available has length restrictions.

SURFACE ANATOMY

The dorsal radial artery is reliably found in the articulation between the proximal metacarpal bones of the thumb and first finger. By superimposing the directional vectors of the thumb and its neighboring finger along the metacarpal bones, their intersection usually signifies the location of the artery, as shown in **Fig. 3**. If one is unable to palpate the artery with ease, it may be too small or deeper than expected. Imaging with vascular ultrasound can quickly answer questions of location and can allow a rapid assessment of the size of the dorsal radial artery. Ultrasound can be used to mark the location of the artery for later puncture or used proactively to guide puncture in real time (**Fig. 4**).

PREPROCEDURE SETUP

The preparatory stage is critical when the operator plans to access the dorsal radial artery. The hand should be rotated in a natural position to maximize exposure to the access site with neither pronation nor supination. The lateral aspect (radial side) of the wrist should be facing up as the patient lays supine. A slight ulnar deviation at the wrist will reduce the angle that the

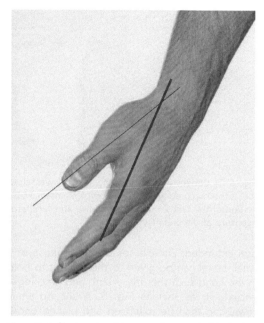

Fig. 3. Left hand with superimposed black line showing vector of the thumb's metacarpal and a red line showing the vector of its neighboring finger's metacarpal. The 2 vectors intersect at the region of where the pulse of the dorsal radial is usually palpable or best seen by ultrasound. This is referred to as the radial apex.

dorsal radial follows as it traverses the base of the thumb and enters the common radial. This position will encourage the wire to pass up the radial artery rather than retroflex down into the palmar arches of the palm.

POSITIONING OF THE WRIST

The patient is placed in the supine position on the catheterization laboratory table with the

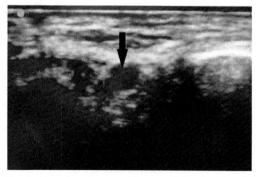

Fig. 4. Vascular ultrasound image of the dorsal radial pointed out with an arrow at the radial apex just beyond the extensor pollicis brevis tendon. Note how the artery lays between the bony structures of snuffbox as if laying in a valley.

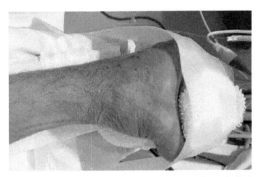

Fig. 5. A patient's hand grasping a small washcloth that is then secured in place. This helps maintain a separation of the first 2 metacarpal bones and facilitates exposure of the underlying artery.

arm extended. Either a roll of 4 × 4 gauze or a small towel can be given to the patient to hold in the hand such that the thumb and first finger encircle it, as seen in Fig. 5. A second small towel can then be rolled up and placed under the ulnar side of the median wrist to give some medial flexion/lateral extension at the wrist that will straighten the dorsal radial course.

A turnkey arm support system (DRAWS Device, Davies Precision Machining, Lebanon, PA) developed by the authors facilitates the positioning for the dorsal radial approach, as shown in Fig. 6. This arm support is designed in a specific fashion to allow easy access to the artery and allow this position to be maintained throughout the procedure. There is a 5° distal angulation that tilts the patient's wrist inferiorly (ulnar wrist flexion). In addition, on the proximal outer portion, there is elbow support (red arrow), and on the distal end of the support, there

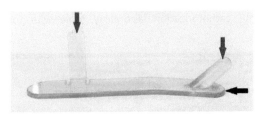

Fig. 6. Arm support board designed by the authors to facilitate positioning for dorsal access at the wrist. This can provide both comfort to the patient and ease to the operator obtaining the access because the arm will lie in the appropriate position and remain stable throughout the position. There is a 5° distal dropdown (black arrow), which will tilt the patient's wrist inferiorly (medial wrist extension). In addition, on the proximal outer portion, there is an elbow support (red arrow), and on the distal region, there is a short rod of Lexan plastic at a 45° angle (blue arrow) that the patient can securely hold during their procedure obviating the need for holding a washcloth.

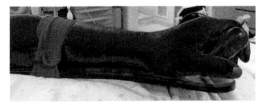

Fig. 7. Arm brace held by patient by the 45° hand mandrel and secured to forearm with an elastic wrap (blue). The arm is then brought to a comfortable working position for access either on the abdomen or on the patient's side depending on operator's preference.

is a mandrel of Lexan plastic that extends at a 45° angle (blue arrow) that the patient can securely hold during their procedure. The forearm is then secured to the arm brace with an elastic bandage while the patient holds on to the 45° plastic mandrel (Fig. 7). As long as the wrist is kept in its medial flexed position, it can be positioned either before or after access with the elbow bent over the patient's abdomen if accessed from the left arm, or remain next to the patient's side in the case of a right arm approach or left arm approach in a thin patient. Different cardiac catheterization laboratories have developed draping preferences, but with the aid of a "donut" and sterile towels the area can be clearly delineated, and a large drape may be then placed over the patient in an aseptic fashion.

ACCESS TECHNIQUE

Once the dorsum of the hand is prepared across the region that encompasses the area overlying the dorsal radial artery, access may be obtained by the use of either ultrasound or palpation, as outlined in Box 1. As seen in Fig. 4, the ultrasonic image at the radial apex just beyond the extensor pollicis brevis tendon shows that the vessel is very superficial and is usually accompanied by one or 2 veins of similar size. The entry technique can be completed in the same manner that the operator is accustomed to whether using a through-and-through technique or the anterior wall puncture technique. The vessel usually lays in a groove with lateral and posterior support from metacarpal structures. Once the vessel is wired, fluoroscopy can be completed to verify the appropriate trajectory seen in Fig. 8, where the wire is seen passing retrograde up the common radial artery. Alternatively, ultrasound of the common radial can also document retrograde passage up the radial. If using a hydrophilic wire, or if resistance is encountered soon after entering the dorsal radial, it is

Box 1
Steps to succeed in dorsal radial access

1. Locate dorsal radial pulse at the base of the thumb and second finger metacarpal bones in the anatomic snuffbox region

2. Position the wrist with thumb side up, slight ulnar flexion to the wrist, and the thumb and neighboring finger separated by a handgrip or towel

3. Vascular ultrasound to confirm the size of vessel and facilitate access

4. Sterile drape of site and access with a micropuncture technique used for radial access

5. Confirm easy passage of wire antegrade up the radial artery

6. Place vascular sheath and complete procedure with usual anticoagulation

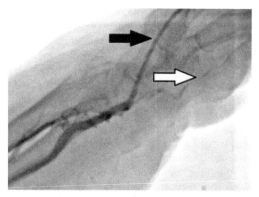

Fig. 9. Angiography through a vascular sheath placed via in the right dorsal radial artery. The black arrow points to the sheath in the dorsal radial and common radial; the white arrow points to the branch that provides blood flow to the palmar arch that remains after the bifurcation of the common radial artery.

possible that the wire has entered the common radial and passed antegrade into the palmar system. If this happens, the operator must withdrawal the wire and reroute it up the forearm. Once sheath placement is secured, upper-extremity angiography may be performed to verify sheath location, as shown in **Fig. 9**. Although routine postsheath placement angiography is not mandatory, it should be used at any point that concerns arise about proper placement or course of the radial arterial system.

Vasodilator cocktails, if used, can be given per local norms, and systemic anticoagulation to minimize the risk of radial artery occlusion should be used after sheath placement. Beyond the nuisances of the sheath placement, the procedure through the dorsal radial artery access site should otherwise be similar to any other typical radial procedure. If a thin-walled sheath is used, care should be taken to prevent kinking across the bend of the dorsal radial as it enters the common radial. Maintaining the wrist in a medially flexed position that straightens the dorsal radial course reduces this tortuosity and the chance for sheath dysfunction.

If the coronary anatomy demonstrates occlusive disease or the need for further evaluation, the sheath may be upsized to accommodate additional equipment or larger guide size. The ability to measure the artery before the procedure is one advantage of using the ultrasound upfront because the operator will already have an idea of vessel size before upsizing. Sheathless guides are an alternative if the diameter of the artery is smaller than desired for traditional sheath approach.

PERCUTANEOUS INTERVENTIONS VIA THE DORSAL RADIAL ARTERY ACCESS

The dorsal radial access can be readily used as an alternative approach in most routine interventions as well as for more difficult procedures, including those with complex coronary disease or chronic total occlusions (CTOs), assuming the individual patient's vessel has sufficient diameter. Also, there is no particular reason it cannot be used for any procedure that requires arterial access, and equipment exists that can reach the intended procedural target.[17] In situations

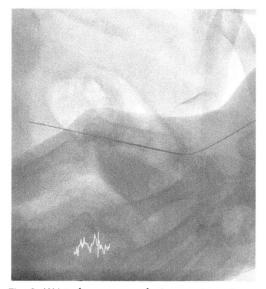

Fig. 8. Wrist after passage of micropuncture wire up arm through an access needle. The wire is seen passing up the artery retrograde rather than taking a sharp turn down into the palm at the junction between the dorsal radial and common radial arteries.

whereby the operator may want left radial access, the left dorsal radial site allows the operator to use the left arm in a position that is comfortable for both the patient and the operator to maintain.

The size of the dorsal radial artery is about 80% of the diameter found in the common radial artery and therefore will in many cases accommodate operators who need larger-bore catheters.[18] A standard 6-French guide catheter will accommodate wires for physiologic testing, intravascular ultrasound, optical coherence testing, workhorse interventions, including orbital or smaller rotational atherectomy devices, trapping balloon, and mother-and-child techniques with most microcatheters. Operators can also consider upsizing to a 7-French or even 8-French Eaucath Sheathless catheter (Asahi Intecc Co, Ltd, Nagoya, Japan), allowing the appropriate inner diameter for most devices, such as orbital or rotational atherectomy, or CrossBoss and Stingray (Boston Scientific, Natick, MA, USA) catheters for antegrade dissection and reentry, and a full range of kissing techniques for complete bifurcation interventions.[19,20] Dual catheters are useful in almost all CTO procedures, and the use of at least one radial artery, if not both, significantly decreases vascular access complications by avoiding the femoral vessels, in addition to improved postprocedural patient comfort. If a decision is made to use bilateral radial artery access for such interventions as CTOs, many operators will use the left radial for their right guide. Access via the dorsal radial offers an approach that may be more comfortable for both the patient and the operator, especially during a lengthy procedure.

Transradial access integrates well with the need for ventricular support devices. Patients on ventricular support devices need large-bore access, and this usually occupies at least one of the femoral arteries. Peripheral vascular disease or concern for access site bleeding may prevent the use of the last remaining femoral site. In these cases, familiarity and experience with a range of forearm access options are essential to adapt the procedure to the patient's situation. Operators who typically prefer the femoral access may choose to use the left radial artery because this access site behaves similarly for them as the femoral artery. It has been noted that left radial artery access has been associated with less catheter manipulation and therefore decreases procedure duration because the catheters, such as Judkins catheters, sit in a similar fashion to a femoral artery because, in both instances, the catheter must be advanced over the aortic arch.[21] Beyond accommodating the needs for coronary intervention, the radial access can also be used for dry closure at the site of large-bore access be it for transcatheter aortic valve replacement or support devices. The radial access can then allow a controlled closure of the femoral arterial puncture without introducing a new femoral puncture and its inherent risks for vascular complications.

POSTPROCEDURE HEMOSTASIS

When the procedure has concluded, the sterile drapes can be removed, leaving the sheath in place (Fig. 10) and the artery ready for hemostasis. Obtaining hemostasis is conceptually similar after dorsal radial artery access compared with standard hemostasis for the common radial artery, but the equipment used is slightly different. The popular hemostasis bands used for the standard radial hemostasis depend on the relative immobility of the distal forearm. Because the distal forearm below the wrist is relatively immobile, hemostatic bands primarily need to work on delivering focused pressure to the access site. The dorsal part of the hand is more mobile because it is located over the wrist bones, and rigid hemostasis devices may be loosened by the patient's wrist movements. A simple and economical solution is the elastic gauze wrap. Use 4 × 4 gauze rolled up tight to form a plug to place at the arterial entry site, as seen in Fig. 11. The gauze placed over the access site

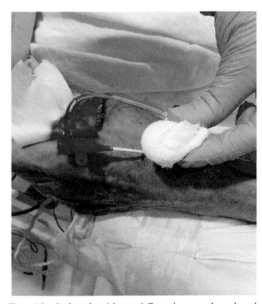

Fig. 10. A hand with a 4-French vascular sheath indwelling the dorsal radial artery after removal of the sterile drapes. Note that the hand is still holding a small washcloth that helps maintain position of the radial apex.

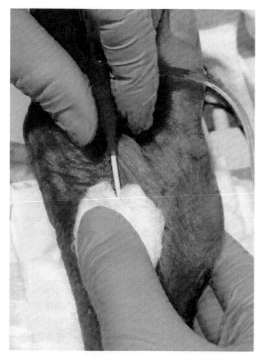

Fig. 11. Vascular sheath removal in progress with 4 × 4 gauze plug ready for external tamponade, later to be supported by elastic bandage.

> **Box 2**
> **Potential indications for dorsal radial access**
>
> 1. Enhance left arm access for patient and physician
> 2. Orthopedic impairment preventing rotation of the arm
> 3. More natural position for a patient to maintain during a lengthy procedure
> 4. Alternative site after recent use of radial access
> 5. Alternative site if other intravenous lines preclude the radial use
> 6. Entry site for retrograde recanalization of radial
> 7. Reduce radial artery injury in the setting of possible future needs

is then wrapped with a tight elastic bandage to tamponade the artery in place, as seen in Video 1. The recovery area staff then observes for hemostasis. The dorsal radial lies in a groove buffered by the wrist bones both below and lateral to each side that appear to facilitate stable hemostasis. The elastic materials tend to loosen with time and often provide a slow release of pressure without interference from the staff, although vigilance to minimize the net pressure and time for hemostasis is prudent. Patent hemostasis that applies just enough pressure to prevent bleeding but not obstruct flow should be attempted where possible, although precise confirmation of antegrade flow may be difficult to determine in this distal access point.

Commercial hemostatic bands that provide some fixation to the site of hemostasis may be useful for the dorsal radial along with modification of other devices. The key is to prevent movement of the point of pressure applied for hemostasis because the underlying wrist bones are moved by the patient. Additional hemostasis bands are being tried to address the challenge of dorsal radial hemostasis.

ADVANTAGES

There are several advantages when it comes to using the dorsal radial artery for access. Some

of the indications for dorsal radial access are noted in **Box 2** and include, most importantly, improved left radial access for both the patient and the operator. The dorsal radial site allows easy access to the radial artery in either arm for patients who have limited arm or shoulder mobility. Even without overt shoulder or elbow injury, the forced rotation at these joints can be painful over a long procedure, especially for the elderly, and the dorsal radial positioning provides a less stressful option. It also allows better ergonomic positioning of the left arm for radial use by the operator, reducing orthopedic stress on the staff encumbered with protective lead.

The dorsal radial artery site also provides a new entry point if the commonly used site has been used recently and is not in an ideal condition to be reused as a result of bruising or hematoma formation. If the radial artery had been previously used, there is a risk that radial artery occlusion has occurred, and the dorsal radial artery access site could provide the operator an ability to recannulate the occluded radial artery, or, likewise, treat a fistula or pseudoaneurysm of the common radial artery.[22] This access site is also located beyond the forearm, which may further reduce the already low risk of compartment syndrome during a radial procedure.

COMPLICATIONS

No particularly unique complications have been reported to date using the dorsal radial access beyond what otherwise might be expected from a standard radial approach. The apparent

Box 3
Potential complications of dorsal radial access

1. Distal embolization

2. Damage to vascular supply of wrist carpal bones (eg, scaphoid bone) that might originate off the dorsal radial

3. Hematoma resulting in compartment syndrome in hand muscle (eg, thenar compartment)

4. Palmar vessel perforation from antegrade wire passage resulting in hematoma

5. Local nerve damage

lack of complications may be the result of underreporting, or perhaps not enough time has elapsed since the introduction of the technique for the true spectrum of potential complications to be seen. Because of the dorsal radial artery's anatomic position and function, several potential complications as noted in **Box 3** may be considered, and operators should be vigilant for their potential appearance.

The most common complication expected would be the inability to do the planned procedure due to the inadequate size of the vessel. A preaccess ultrasound is the best protection against this occurrence because the size of the vessel can be accurately assessed, and an informed decision can be made regarding the adequacy of the vessel for potential procedures. From common experience, it appears that about 20% of the population may not have a dorsal radial vessel adequate in size for cardiac catheterization procedures.

Radial artery occlusion remains a problem for both dorsal and traditional radial access points. Contributing factors include trauma from vessel wall puncture at the site of vascular sheath entry along with vessel wall dissection and deendothelialization from direct trauma by the passage of the vascular sheath.[23] Limiting trauma to the vessel by first stick techniques, use of anticoagulation, postprocedure antispasm medications,[24,25] and patent hemostasis can minimize, although not eliminate, the rate of radial artery occlusion.[2] Fortunately, in the short run, this complication is asymptomatic, although over the longer term, it precludes the further use of that radial artery.

Initial series of dorsal radial access have shown an interesting pattern for radial occlusion.[10–12] Occlusion rates appear on par with that observed following best practice with the standard radial approach, but the site of occlusion remains

primarily in the dorsal segment with only a minority extending into the primary radial channel. This pattern of radial occlusion may be due to the protection against sheath trauma in the larger radial vessel because the size of the dorsal branch limits the size of the sheath used, and therefore, less vascular wall trauma may extend into the radial artery. Another explanation may be that during hemostasis, flow may be occluded or reduced in the dorsal radial artery at the site of sheath entry, but normal flow remains in the common radial, thereby protecting that vessel from low-flow thrombosis. Further observations are needed, and approaches that further reduce radial thrombosis whether in the common or dorsal branch of the radial artery are still to be elucidated.

SUMMARY

The dorsal radial artery presents a unique access site that may ultimately improve options for operators and patients. This technique is a relatively novel technique vetted primarily on social media and by a few small single-center experiences. It appears to offer improvement in the radial catheterization experience for patients who are orthopedically challenged by the positioning required for traditional transradial access. The added flexibility of the access site also improves the ergonomics for the operator. Whether distal radial access provides a potential benefit of reduced radial artery occlusion, or the specter of hand muscle compartment syndromes and wrist bone avascular necrosis, requires further exploration.

VIDEO

Video related to this article can be found online at https://doi.org/10.1016/j.iccl.2018.11.002

REFERENCES

1. Davies RE, Gilchrist IC. Back hand approach to radial access: the snuff box approach. Cardiovasc Revasc Med 2018;19:324–6. Available at: https://www.sciencedirect.com/science/article/pii/S1553838917303366?via=ihub.

2. Caputo RP, Tremmel JA, Rao S, et al. Transradial arterial access for coronary and peripheral procedures: executive summary by the transradial committee of the SCAI. Catheter Cardiovasc Interv 2011; 78(6):823–39.

3. Amato JJ, Solod E, Cleveland RJ. A "second" radial artery for monitoring the perioperative pediatric cardiac patient. J Pediatr Surg 1977;12(5): 715–7.

4. Pyles ST, Scher KS, Vega ET, et al. Cannulation of the dorsal radial artery: a new technique. Anesth Analg 1982;61:876–8.
5. Moore KP. Cannulation of the dorsal radial artery. Anesth Analg 1983;62(5):540.
6. Tibbetts TM. Dorsal continuation of the radial artery. Can J Anaesth 2002;49:438–40.
7. Deepika K, Palaniappan D, Fuhrman T, et al. Anatomic snuffbox radial artery cannulation. Anesth Analg 2010;111(4):1078–9. Available at: https://journals.lww.com/anesthesia-analgesia/Full-text/2010/10000/Anatomic_Snuffbox_Radial_Artery_Cannulation.50.aspx.
8. Kimura Y, Kimura S, Inoue H, et al. Comparison of usefulness of the dorsal branch of the radial artery with the radial artery for arterial cannulation. Masui 2012;61(7):728–32. Available at: https://www.ncbi.nlm.nih.gov/pubmed/22860301.
9. Choi S, Park J-M, Nam SH, et al. Cannulation of the dorsal radial artery: an underused, yet useful, technique. Korean J Anesthesiol 2014;67(Suppl):S11–2. Available at: https://ekja.org/journal/view.php?doi=10.4097/kjae.2014.67.S.S11.
10. Kaledin AL, Kochanov IN, Podmetin PS, et al. Distal radial artery in endovascular interventions. Research 2017. https://doi.org/10.13140/RG.2.2.13406.33600. Available at: https://www.research-gate.net/publication/319162208. Accessed August 15, 2018.
11. Kiemeneij F. Left distal transradial access in the anatomical snuffbox for coronary angiography (ldTRA) and interventions (ldTRI). EuroIntervention 2017;13(7):851–7. Available at: https://www.pcronline.com/eurointervention/122nd_issue/volume-13/number-7/124/left-distal-transradial-access-in-the-anatomical-snuffbox-for-coronary-angiography-ldtra-and-interventions-ldtri.html.
12. Amin MR, Singha CK, Banerjee SK, et al. Comparison of distal transradial in the anatomical suffbox versus conventional transradial access for coronary angiography and intervention- an experience in 100 cases. University Heart Journal 2017;13(2):40–5. Available at: https://www.banglajol.info/index.php/UHJ/article/view/37657.
13. Soydan E, Akin M. Coronary angiography using the left distal radial approach – An alternative site to conventional radial coronary angiography. Anatol J Cardiol 2018;19:243–8. Available at: http://www.anakarder.com/jvi.aspx?pdir=anatoljcardiol&plng=eng&un=AJC-59932.
14. Valsecchi O, Vassileva A, Cereda AF, et al. Early clinical experience with right and left distal transradial access in the anatomical snuffbox in 52 consecutive patients. J Invasive Cardiol 2018;30(6):218–23. Available at: https://www.invasivecardiology.com/articles/early-clinical-experience-right-and-left-distal-transradial-access-anatomical-snuffbox-52.
15. Roghani-Dehkordi F, Hashemifard O, Sadeghi M, et al. Distal accesses in the hand (two novel techniques) for percutaneous coronary angiography and intervention. ARYA Atheroscler 2018;14(2):95–100.
16. Hull JE, Kinsey EN, Bishop WL. Mapping of the snuffbox and cubital vessels for percutaneous arterial venous fistula (pAVF) in dialysis patients. J Vasc Access 2013;14:245–51.
17. Pua U, Sim JZT, Quek LHH, et al. Feasibility study of "snuffbox" radial access for visceral interventions. J Vasc Interv Radiol 2018;29(9):1276–80.
18. Gilchrist IC, Awuor S, Davies RE, et al. Controversies in complex percutaneous coronary intervention: radial versus femoral. Expert Rev Cardiovasc Ther 2017;15(9):695–704.
19. Dautov R, Ribeiro HB, Abdul-Jawad Altisent O, et al. Effectiveness and safety of the transradial 8Fr sheathless approach for revascularization of chronic total occlusions. Am J Cardiol 2016;118:785–9.
20. Rinfret S, Joyal D, Spratt JC, et al. Chronic total occlusion percutaneous coronary intervention case selection and techniques for the antegrade-only operator. Catheter Cardiovasc Interv 2015;85:408–15.
21. Kawashima O, Endoh N, Terashima M, et al. Effectiveness of right or left radial approach for coronary angiography. Catheter Cardiovasc Interv 2004;61:333–7.
22. Babunashvili AM, Pancholy SB, Kartashov DS. New technique for treatment of postcatheterization radial artery pseudoaneurysm. Catheter Cardiovasc Interv 2017;89(3):393–8.
23. Yonetsu T, Kakuta T, Lee T, et al. Assessment of acute injuries and chronic intimal thickening of the radial artery after transradial coronary intervention by optical coherence tomography. Eur Heart J 2010;31(13):1608–15.
24. Dharma S, Kedev S, Patel T, et al. A novel approach to reduce radial artery occlusion after transradial catheterization: postprocedural/prehemostasis intra-arterial nitroglycerin. Catheter Cardiovasc Interv 2015;85(5):818–25.
25. Chen Y, Ke Z, Xiao J, et al. Subcutaneous injection of nitroglycerin at the radial artery puncture site reduces the risk of early radial artery occlusion after transradial coronary catheterization: a randomized, placebo-controlled clinical trial. Circ Cardiovasc Interv 2018;11:e006571.

Clinical Outcomes Data for Instantaneous Wave-Free Ratio-Guided Percutaneous Coronary Intervention

Masood Younus, MD[a], Arnold H. Seto, MD, MPA[a,b],*

KEYWORDS

• iFR • PCI outcomes • Instantaneous wave-free ratio

KEY POINTS

- Instantaneous wave-free ratio (iFR) is a vasodilator-free index of coronary blood flow used to aid in decision-making for revascularization.
- iFR-SWEDEHEART and DEFINE-FLAIR were 2 large randomized controlled trials that demonstrated the noninferiority of iFR compared with fractional-flow reserve (FFR) for major adverse cardiac events.
- These studies showed several advantages of iFR, including lack of adverse effects from vasodilators, shorter procedure times, and lower rates of revascularization without increased MACE.
- iFR-pullback may be useful to assess tandem and diffuse coronary disease in revascularization planning.
- iFR may be particularly useful in patients with potential adenosine resistance, contraindications to adenosine, and multivessel or serial lesions; it may be used with or without FFR for revascularization planning.

INTRODUCTION

Revascularization through percutaneous coronary intervention (PCI) improves symptoms in patients with coronary artery disease (CAD) and improves morbidity and mortality in patients with acute coronary syndromes (ACS). Coronary angiography guides revascularization based solely on the angiographic appearance of stenoses relative to the reference vessel and is limited in predicting the physiologic impact of a stenosis.

Over the past 20-plus years, the superiority of physiologic guidance of revascularization decisions over angiography alone has been demonstrated across multiple studies. Preliminary work demonstrated the utility and safety of deferring PCI in coronary lesions with low-risk coronary hemodynamics.[1,2] Fractional-flow reserve (FFR) emerged as a standardized index of coronary flow hemodynamics that has useful clinical applications without the technical challenges and variability of direct flow measurements.[3] FFR represents the ratio of the maximal blood flow to the myocardium supplied by a coronary artery in the presence of stenosis (Pd) compared with the theoretic maximal blood flow (Pa) in the absence of the stenosis. Intracoronary or intravenous adenosine is used to induce hyperemia in the coronary vessel, and the ratio between Pd and Pa is measured during maximal hyperemia. Although

Disclosure Statement: Dr A. Seto has received research grants and honoraria from Philips.

[a] Department of Medicine, University of California, 101 The City Drive South, Orange, CA 92868, USA;
[b] Department of Medicine, Veterans Administration Long Beach Health Care System, 5901 East 7th Street, 111C, Long Beach, CA 90822, USA
* Corresponding author. Department of Medicine, Veterans Administration Long Beach Health Care System, 5901 East 7th Street, 111C, Long Beach, CA 90822.
E-mail address: aseto@uci.edu

a Pd/Pa ratio of less than or equal to 0.74 was identified as a cutoff for coronary stenosis causing ischemia,[4] a cutoff of less than or equal to 0.8 emerged as the clinical standard. Outcomes data based on the large DEFER,[5] FAME (Fractional Flow Reserve vs Angiography for Multivessel Evaluation),[6] FAME II,[7] and RIPCORD[8] trials convincingly demonstrated improved patient outcomes with FFR-guided PCI, offering prognostic and symptomatic advantages to medical therapy, whereas PCI of nonsignificant stenosis does not.

Despite this abundance of evidence for FFR-guided PCI, which eventually led to a class I guideline recommendation for using FFR for the assessment of intermediate-grade stenosis,[9] adoption rates of FFR have been poor.[10] This is likely due to a combination of factors, but especially the requirement for adenosine administration. Adenosine infusion in the catheterization laboratory requires trained nursing personnel, carries additional costs, and can result in patient discomfort, arrhythmias, and bronchospasm.

The instantaneous wave-free ratio (iFR), a vasodilator-free methodology for evaluating coronary hemodynamics for PCI, was derived from the FFR concept while overcoming the requirement of induced hyperemia. This resting pressure index measures coronary pressures across the coronary stenosis during a "wave-free" period in diastole where microvascular resistance is naturally relatively low and stable. This resting pressure index correlates with reasonable (80%) accuracy with pressures measured during hyperemic FFR.[11] Multiple follow-up studies[12–15] demonstrated concordance of iFR and FFR for assessing coronary stenosis severity and established an iFR of less than 0.90 (or $\leq$0.89) as the best cut-off for treatment based on its correlation with the standard of FFR less than or equal to 0.80.

The ADVISE (Vasodilator Free Measure of Fractional Flow Reserve)-II cohort study[14] established the validity of iFR and proposed a hybrid iFR-FFR approach to increase accuracy of diagnosis, and a recent meta-analysis assessing the validity of iFR compared with FFR over 16 studies and 5756 lesions found a diagnostic accuracy of 81%.[16] However, some studies such as the VERIFY (VERification of Instantaneous Wave-Free Ratio and Fractional Flow Reserve for the Assessment of Coronary Artery Stenosis Severity in EverydaY Practice)[17] and VERIFY II trials[18] challenge the idea that nonhyperemic indices of stenosis such as iFR have the same accuracy as FFR and may lead to significant lesion misclassification.

The potential for iFR to improve utilization of physiology-based PCI due to shorter procedural times, decreased costs, and decreased patient side effects compared with FFR was appreciated by some, but clinical outcome studies measuring hard clinical endpoints such as major adverse cardiac events (MACE) were needed to determine the true safety and efficacy of iFR-guided PCI. This article reviews the existing outcomes data for iFR, provides context for its place in guiding PCI, highlights where additional clinical outcome data is needed, and outlines directions for future studies.

RANDOMIZED CLINICAL TRIALS
DEFINE-FLAIR

The DEFINE-FLAIR (Functional Lesion Assessment of Intermediate Stenosis to Guide Revascularization)[19] trial was a randomized, international, multicenter, blinded trial that aimed to determine if iFR was noninferior to FFR in terms of MACE at 1-year follow-up. Patients included in the study had CAD and either stable angina or ACS with at least one native coronary vessel with "questionable physiologic severity," defined as 40% to 70% stenosis by visual, angiographic assessment. Patients were excluded if they had tandem stenoses separated by more than 10 mm, restenotic lesions, left main stenosis greater than 50%, total coronary occlusions, heavy calcification, prior coronary artery bypass grafting (CABG), or several other comorbid conditions. A total of 2492 patients were randomized to have revascularization guided by either iFR (1242 patients) or FFR (1250 patients) but not both (in contrast to prior correlation studies). The patient and follow-up caregivers were also blinded to the group assignment. The prespecified PCI treatment threshold for FFR was less than or equal to 0.80 and iFR less than or equal to 0.89. The measured primary outcome was MACE, a composite of death, nonfatal myocardial infarction (MI), or unplanned revascularization. The noninferiority margin was prespecified as a 3.4% difference in risk, based on an assumed annual rate of 8.5%, in line with other major cardiovascular outcome trials.

Procedural characteristics differed between iFR and FFR with respect to median procedure time (40.5 min vs 45.0 min respectively, $P<.001$, number of functionally significant lesions evaluated (451 [28.6%] vs 557 [38.9%], $P = .004$), more than or equal to 1 functionally significant lesions (426 [34.3%] vs 486 [38.9%], $P = .02$), and total revascularizations performed (590 [47.5%] vs 667 [53.4%], $P = .003$). There was a significantly higher frequency of patient-reported adverse procedural symptoms or signs in the FFR group versus the iFR group (385 [30.8%] vs 39 [3.1%], respectively, $P<.001$) due to the use of intravenous adenosine, including bronchospasm and ventricular arrhythmias in 8 patients in the FFR group. These data are consistent with prior studies that demonstrated a higher rate of adverse effects with FFR.

The primary endpoint of MACE was not significantly different between the iFR group and the FFR group, with difference in risk of −0.2 percentage points (95% confidence interval [CI] −2.3–1.8 vs 95% CI −2.9–2.5 respectively, $P = .83$). The hazard ratio for MACE with iFR was 0.95 (95% CI 0.68–1.33, $P = .78$). Fig. 1 is a Kaplan–Meier curve demonstrating the noninferiority of iFR for the primary endpoint. The individual component endpoints of unplanned revascularization ($P = .13$), nonfatal MI ($P = .62$), death from cardiovascular causes ($P = .34$), death from noncardiovascular causes ($P = .34$), and death from any cause ($P = .11$) were also not significantly different. These findings were confirmed in the subsequent, more stringent per-protocol analysis, which demonstrated a hazard ratio of 0.94 (95% CI 0.67–1.31, $P = .82$) and risk difference of −0.3 percentage points in iFR versus FFR (95% CI −2.4–1.8 vs 95% CI −3.0–2.4 respectively, $P = .77$).

These data demonstrated that iFR-based PCI was noninferior to FFR-based PCI. Although iFR assessment led to less revascularization with both PCI and CABG compared with FFR, there was no significant difference in MACE, in both the intention-to-treat and the per-protocol analysis groups.

Instantaneous Wave-Free Ratio-SWEDEHEART

The iFR-SWEDEHEART (Instantaneous Wave-free Ratio Versus Fractional Flow Reserve in Patients with Stable Angina Pectoris or Acute Coronary Syndrome) trial was the second large study in 2017 directly comparing clinical outcomes between FFR and iFR.[20] As with DEFINE-FLAIR, this was a multicenter, randomized, controlled, clinical trial but used a Swedish registry for enrollment and data collection and was thus open-label. Patients with stable angina, unstable angina, or prior non-ST elevation MI with indications for physiologically guided assessment of CAD (40%–80% stenosis on visual examination) were enrolled. All lesions were evaluated in patients with stable angina; nonculprit lesions were measured in patients with unstable angina or non-ST elevation MI. A total of 2037 patients across 15 hospitals in Sweden, Denmark, and Iceland were enrolled into the trial with 1019 in the iFR group and 1018 in the FFR group. The PCI treatment threshold for FFR was less than or equal to 0.80 and for iFR was less than or equal to 0.89. The primary endpoint was the composite rate of all-cause death, nonfatal MI, or unplanned revascularization within 12 months after intervention. Secondary endpoints were the individual component rates of the primary end point, chest discomfort during the procedure, target lesion revascularization, stent thrombosis, and restenosis. The study was powered for a noninferiority margin of 3.2% between treatments, which was equal to a hazard ratio of 1.40.

The iFR and FFR groups were similar in baseline characteristics and demographics. The mean iFR was 0.91 ± 0.10, and the mean FFR was 0.82 ± 0.10. The iFR group had significantly more lesions evaluated per patient compared with the FFR group (1.55 ± 0.86 vs 1.43 ± 0.70, $P = .002$). However, as in DEFINE-FLAIR, there were significantly fewer hemodynamically significant lesions as assessed by iFR compared with FFR (29.1% vs 36.8%, $P<.001$), leading to a fewer stents placed per patient (1.58 ± 1.08 vs 1.73 ± 1.19, $P = .05$).

The primary endpoint occurred in 6.7% in the iFR group compared with 6.1% in the FFR group, as shown in. The difference in event rates between treatments was 0.7% (95% CI of −1.5–2.8, $P = .007$ for noninferiority), which corresponds to a hazard ratio of 1.12 (95% CI 0.79–1.58, $P = .53$). There were 15 deaths in the iFR group compared with 12 in the FFR group. The rates of all other component secondary endpoints did not differ significantly between groups. Chest discomfort during the procedure differed significantly between the 2 groups, with 3.0% in the iFR group versus 68.3% in the FFR group ($P = .001$), due to adenosine use.

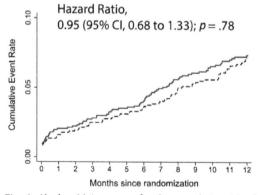

Hazard Ratio, 0.95 (95% CI, 0.68 to 1.33); $p = .78$

Fig. 1. Kaplan–Meier curves for the cumulative risk of the primary endpoint of the DEFINE-FLAIR clinical trial (composite of death from any cause, nonfatal myocardial infarction, or unplanned revascularization) at 1 year in patients treated with FFR (*red*) and iFR (*black*). (*From* Davies J, Sen S, Dehbi H, et al. Use of the instantaneous wave-free ratio or fractional flow reserve in PCI. N Engl J Med 2017;376(19):1832, as adapted by Dr Justin Davies; with permission.)

The authors of the study noted that more lesions were assessed in the iFR group than FFR, which may have occurred because of the greater chest discomfort seen with FFR, decreasing the assessment of subsequent nonculprit lesions. The authors postulate that this difference is not likely to have influenced outcomes because rates of death and MI are low in FFR values close to 0.80, based on a prospective study[21] in 2016. In addition, there may have been an overestimation of clinically significant lesions using the clinical threshold of 0.80 rather than 0.75. Some limitations to this study noted by the authors include the generous noninferiority margin of 40% relative risk, combined with the overall low primary endpoint event rates observed for both iFR and FFR. In addition, group assignments were not blinded to physicians and patients, which may have affected decisions for revascularization.

Pooled Analyses

The iFR-SWEDEHEART and DEFINE-FLAIR studies were designed to have similar designs and endpoints to facilitate a pooled analysis. Across both studies, PCI was deferred more frequently in the iFR group compared with the FFR group (50% vs 45%, $P<.01$). At 1 year, the MACE rate in the deferred population was similar between the iFR and FFR groups (4.12% vs 4.05%; fully adjusted hazard ratio, 1.13; 95% CI, 0.72–1.79; $P = .60$).[22]

Berry and colleagues[23] compared rates of death and MI between the FFR and iFR groups in the 2 trials using risk ratios derived from published data. Rates of death, nonfatal MI, and unplanned revascularization were statistically nonsignificant with P-values greater than 0.05. Of the 160 deaths or MI events in 4345 patients observed at the 12-month follow-up, 90 were in the iFR group and 70 were in the FFR group, resulting in a numeric but nonsignificant excess in death or MI in patients in the iFR group (hazard ratio 1.30, 95% CI 0.96–1.77, $P = .09$). Berry and colleagues argued that although the lower limit of the CI crossed unity, the upper limit of the 95% CI indicates that "risk for adverse outcome could be $\leq77\%$ greater for iFR guidance compared with FFR guidance." These authors suggest iFR may in fact be inferior to FFR for clinical outcomes, given the numerical excess of events in the pooled iFR group, the lack of blinding in iFR-SWEDEHEART, and the lower power to detect a difference between groups because of the inherent concordance of 80% between FFR and iFR and the overall lower risk population enrolled. This analysis is

appropriately concerned with the more serious clinical outcomes of death or MI compared with revascularization but remains a post hoc selection of specific outcomes with inherent limitations.

NONRANDOMIZED STUDIES
3V FFR-FRIENDS

Both DEFINE-FLAIR and iFR-SWEDEHEART sorted patients into exclusively iFR- or FFR-guided groups. No prior study had assessed the outcomes of patients with discordant FFR and iFR results. A substudy of the 3V FFR-FRIENDS (3-Vessel Fractional Flow Reserve for the Assessment of Total Stenosis Burden and Its Clinical Impact in Patients with Coronary Artery Disease) study investigated 2-year outcomes in patients with deferred lesions where both iFR and FFR were measured.[24] This substudy was performed across 4 centers and included 374 patients with 821 deferred lesions. The primary outcome was MACE, defined as cardiac death, MI, and ischemia-driven revascularization. The cutoff for physiological significance was less than or equal to 0.80 for FFR and less than or equal to 0.89 for iFR, but revascularization was performed according to operator discretion. Patients were classified into 4 groups: concordant normal, high FFR and low iFR, low FFR and high iFR, and concordant abnormal. Analysis of 2-year outcomes was performed in a blinded manner on a per-patient and per-vessel basis.

Lesions with concordant low FFR and low iFR findings had significantly higher stenosis severity and length compared with lesions with high FFR and high iFR findings, respectively. Patients with low FFR or low iFR lesions for whom revascularization was deferred had significantly (5-fold) higher rates of MACE compared with high FFR (7.2% vs 2.4%, $P<.001$) and high iFR (8.1% vs 2.4%, $P<.001$), respectively. FFR and iFR were equivalent in predicting adverse outcomes, with a c-index 0.677 and 0.685 ($P = .857$), respectively.

Rates of MACE were compared between the 4 groups of lesions (Fig. 2). Only the concordant abnormal FFR/iFR group had a significantly higher rate of MACE compared with the concordant normal group, whereas the discordant groups did not have a significantly higher rate of events. The implication is that among patients with lesions that are FFR+/iFR– or FFR–/iFR+ for ischemia, the clinical event rate is not clearly worse compared with concordant normal lesions. This supports the concept that iFR is noninferior to FFR and that in cases of FFR/iFR

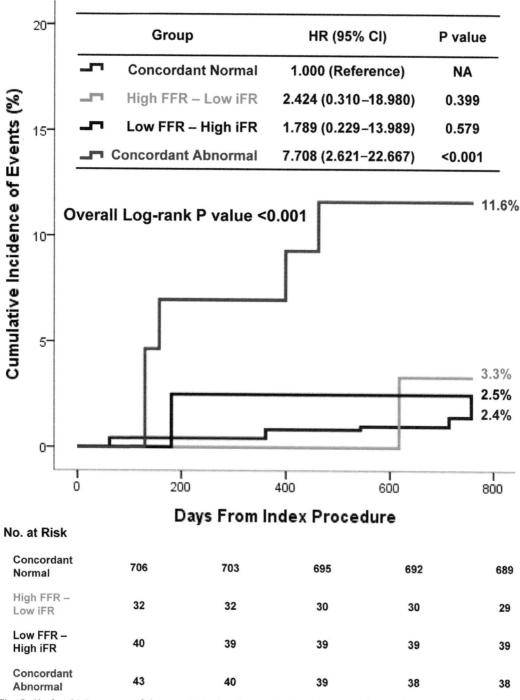

Group	HR (95% CI)	P value
Concordant Normal	1.000 (Reference)	NA
High FFR – Low iFR	2.424 (0.310–18.980)	0.399
Low FFR – High iFR	1.789 (0.229–13.989)	0.579
Concordant Abnormal	7.708 (2.621–22.667)	<0.001

Overall Log-rank P value <0.001

No. at Risk

Concordant Normal	706	703	695	692	689
High FFR – Low iFR	32	32	30	30	29
Low FFR – High iFR	40	39	39	39	39
Concordant Abnormal	43	40	39	38	38

Fig. 2. Kaplan–Meier curves of the cumulative incidence of major adverse cardiovascular events after deferral of lesions according to 4 categories based on FFR and iFR. The concordant abnormal group was the only group with a significantly higher cumulative incidence of events compared with the other groups. (*From* Lee J, Shin E, Nam C, et al. Clinical outcomes according to fractional flow reserve or instantaneous wave-free ratio in deferred lesions. JACC Cardiovasc Interv 2017;10(24):2506; with permission.)

discordance, an isolated iFR+ or FFR+ measurement may overestimate the ischemic potential of a lesion and the consequences of deferral. Because FFR less than 0.80 more frequently identifies lesions as requiring revascularization (by 10% in DEFINE-FLAIR and IFR-SWEDE HEART), and FFR+/iFR-is more frequently encountered than FFR−/iFR+, FFR may be more likely to overestimate lesion significance than iFR. Conceptually, this may be because of higher than expected flow rates during hyperemia that create lower FFR values across lesions that have minimal resting gradients.

Limitations of this study include a small number of MACE events in total, a predominantly low-risk population (average FFR was 0.90%, and 89.9% of lesions had FFR >0.80), and a lack of difference in cardiac death or vessel-related MI. These limitations likely underpowered the study's ability to detect differences in MACE between the 2 modalities.

SYNTAX II

The SYNTAX II (A Trial to Evaluate a New Strategy in the Functional Assessment of 3-Vessel Disease Using the SYNTAX II Score in Patients Treated with PCI) study[25] demonstrated a possible application of using an iFR-FFR hybrid approach to determine revascularization decision-making using FFR when iFR is found to be in an intermediate range (0.86–0.93). The SYNTAX Score II is a clinical tool that combines anatomic and clinical factors to aid in decision-making between CABG and PCI based on 4-year mortality. In this multicenter, open label, single-arm study in patients with multivessel disease, patients had the severity of their coronary lesions objectively characterized with the SYNTAX score II to decide between revascularization strategies. Major adverse cardiac and cerebrovascular events were evaluated at 1 year. All suitable lesions (1177/1338) were evaluated with physiologic indices regardless of angiographic severity, and iFR was used in 1150 (73.8%) cases. Most of the lesions with iFR less than 0.86 (n = 603, 52.4%) were treated (n = 600), whereas most of the lesions with iFR greater than 0.93 (n = 283, 24.6%) were deferred (n = 262). Lesions with intermediate iFR (n = 264, 23%) had a subsequent FFR measurement resulting in 179 treated lesions and 85 deferred lesions. The use of the SYNTAX score II and the "hybrid approach" of FFR measurements in intermediate range iFR lesions may provide operators with an additional tool to plan revascularization in patients with multivessel disease.

DEFINE-REAL

Although the studies discussed earlier measured clinical outcomes of iFR-guided PCI, the DEFINE-REAL trial studied the effect of iFR data on clinical decision-making in patients with multivessel disease.[26] In a total of 484 patients with multivessel disease, 828 out of 1097

vessels interrogated by angiography were investigated with invasive physiology, either by FFR (n = 324 patients) or by iFR (n = 160). In addition to confirming the high agreement between iFR and FFR (92%), this prospective observational study showed that routine invasive physiology with FFR or iFR led to a high rate of lesion reclassification (26%) and overall management reclassification (45%) compared with the original revascularization strategy based on angiographic guidance. The use of iFR was associated with the interrogation of more vessels (P = .04) compared with FFR and a higher overall management reclassification rate compared (57.5% vs 39.9%, P = .0001), without an increase in the rate of major periprocedural safety events. This study confirms in a clinical observational study that the ease of iFR measurement facilitates and encourages the measurement of multiple vessels. Compared with FFR, IFR reclassified a larger number of patients from their original angiographic strategy, although the clinical benefit of higher reclassification rates is unclear.

Instantaneous Wave-Free Ratio-GRADIENT

iFR-GRADIENT (Single Instantaneous Wave-free Ratio Pullback Pre-angioplasty Predicts Hemodynamic Outcome Without Wedge Pressure in Human Coronary Artery Disease) was a multicenter trial that examined the performance of in-line iFR-pullback in serial and diffuse lesions to predict physiologic outcomes post-PCI[27] (Fig. 3). A total of 159 patients with 168 coronary vessels indicated for PCI were enrolled. Post-PCI iFR was predicted from the iFR gradient across the lesions to be treated and distal pre-PCI iFR measured at the distal coronary artery. The predicted post-PCI iFR correlated well with the observed post-PCI iFR (0.93 ± 0.05 vs 0.92 ± 0.06, r = 0.73, P<.001), with an average difference of 1.4%. Compared with conventional angiography alone, the addition of real-time iFR-pullback data changed revascularization planning in 43 of 159 (30%) patients and 52 of 168 (31%) vessels. There was a significant decrease in the number (P = .0001) and length (P<.0001) of hemodynamically significant lesions planned for revascularization. The high accuracy of the post-PCI iFR prediction is in contrast to FFR measurements of serial lesions, because resting flow tends to be constant following PCI of a single lesion, whereas the increased flow with adenosine following PCI of one lesion can increase the gradient of non-stented lesions (cross-talk) in a manner that is difficult to predict. This concept is demonstrated in Fig. 4.

A iFR is Calculated as the Ratio of Pd to Pa on a Beat-by-beat Basis

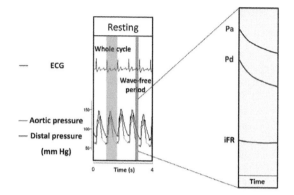

B iFR Pullback for Quantification of Lesion Severity

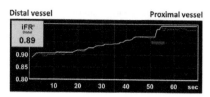

C Procedural Planning and the Prediction of Post-PCI iFR Outcome

Using iFR pullback data, the operators planned the procedure and predicted and registered iFR outcome into an electronic case report form before starting PCI. iFR was predicted by summation of iFR gradient and iFR measured at the distal coronary artery before treatment procedure (**B, C**: red bar).

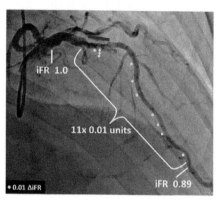

Fig. 3. Prediction of post-PCI physiology based on pre-PCI iFR-pullback across serial lesions. (*A*) Pre-PCI iFR was measured during the wave-free period of diastole. (*B*) iFR-pullback was used to quantify lesion severity across serial lesions. (*C*) Post-PCI iFR was predicted using pre-PCI iFR gradient summation (*yellow dots*) and the iFR measured distally. Intervention planning was done using these data (*red bar*). (*From* Kikuta Y, Cook C, Sharp A, et al. Pre-angioplasty instantaneous wave-free ratio pullback predicts hemodynamic outcome in humans with coronary artery disease. JACC Cardiovasc Interv 2018;11(8):759; with permission.)

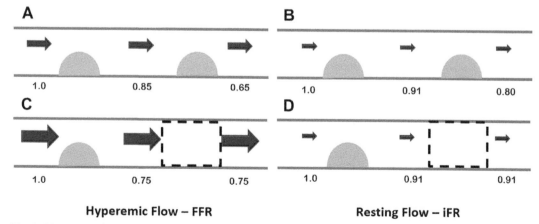

Hyperemic Flow – FFR **Resting Flow – iFR**

Fig. 4. Measuring physiologic severity of serial lesions with iFR compared with FFR. FFR measurements before PCI of the distant vessel (*A*) imply that only the distal lesion is physiologically significant (≤0.80), but after PCI the proximal lesion FFR measurement becomes significant (*C*). In contrast, pre-PCI iFR (*B*) and post-PCI iFR (*D*) of the proximal lesion are consistent and physiologically insignificant (>0.90) due to unchanged resting flow.

Taken together, these studies suggest that the real-time assessment of coronary lesion hemodynamics with iFR, which has the added advantage of being accurate in tandem and diffuse lesions, leads to significant changes in revascularization planning. Although lacking clinical outcomes data, these trials project exciting new directions for the utility of iFR.

SUMMARY

The studies reviewed herein represent the presently available trials with outcomes data for iFR. The discordance observed between FFR and iFR, which seems to occur in approximately 8% to 20% of cases, does not seem to translate into a significant difference in clinical outcomes. Although there have been several studies evaluating FFR over many years, the number of patients collectively enrolled in iFR trials (n = 5972) far outnumber the total enrollment of the DEFER, FAME, and FAME-2 studies. This supports the concept that iFR-guided PCI is safe, noninferior to FFR for clinical outcomes, eliminates adenosine-related costs and adverse effects, and is potentially more efficient in directing revascularization toward patients at risk of MACE.

The optimal choice between FFR and iFR for physiologic assessment may be situation-dependent. Some patients are poorly tolerant of adenosine (eg, those with conduction system disease or at risk of bronchospasm), whereas others may have an attenuated response to adenosine (eg, coffee drinkers; those with microvascular disease, diabetes, dialysis, or recent ACS), where an adenosine-free index of physiologic assessment would be preferred. In time-sensitive cases, when multiple vessels need interrogation, and when there are diffuse or tandem lesions, iFR may more efficiently and precisely localize the area of stenosis requiring treatment. Conversely, iFR may underestimate the ischemic potential of coronary lesions in the left main and left anterior descending lesions where flow is highest.[28]

Usually, a single test will be positive enough to guide decisions; however, in borderline cases where both indices are available, it may be prudent to measure both FFR and iFR to justify revascularization decisions. It is reassuring that to the best of the authors' current knowledge, iFR seems to perform as well as FFR in guiding revascularization, and long-term follow-up outcomes of the DEFINE-FLAIR and iFR-SWEDEHEART trials may provide further support for this conclusion. For now, there are 2 equally powerful tools to guide operators in revascularization decision-making.

REFERENCES

1. Kern M, Donohue T, Aguirre F, et al. Clinical outcome of deferring angioplasty in patients with normal translesional pressure-flow velocity measurements. J Am Coll Cardiol 1995;25(1):178–87.

2. Serruys P, di Mario C, Piek J, et al. Prognostic value of intracoronary flow velocity and diameter stenosis in assessing the short- and long-term outcomes of coronary balloon angioplasty : the DEBATE Study (Doppler endpoints balloon angioplasty trial Europe). Circulation 1997;96(10):3369–77.

3. Pijls N, van Son J, Kirkeeide R, et al. Experimental basis of determining maximum coronary, myocardial, and collateral blood flow by pressure measurements for assessing functional stenosis severity before and after percutaneous transluminal coronary angioplasty. Circulation 1993;87(4):1354–67.

4. Pijls N, Van Gelder B, Van der Voort P, et al. Fractional flow reserve : a useful index to evaluate the influence of an epicardial coronary stenosis on myocardial blood flow. Circulation 1995;92(11):3183–93.

5. Pijls N, van Schaardenburgh P, Manoharan G, et al. Percutaneous coronary intervention of functionally nonsignificant stenosis. J Am Coll Cardiol 2007;49(21):2105–11.

6. Tonino P, De Bruyne B, Pijls N, et al. Fractional flow reserve versus angiography for guiding percutaneous coronary intervention. N Engl J Med 2009;360(3):213–24.

7. De Bruyne B, Pijls N, Kalesan B, et al. Fractional flow reserve–guided PCI versus medical therapy in stable coronary disease. N Engl J Med 2012;367(11):991–1001.

8. Curzen N, Rana O, Nicholas Z, et al. Does routine pressure wire assessment influence management strategy at coronary angiography for diagnosis of chest pain?: the RIPCORD study. Circ Cardiovasc Interv 2014;7(2):248–55.

9. Neumann F, Sousa-Uva M, Ahlsson A, et al. 2018 ESC/EACTS Guidelines on myocardial revascularization. Eur Heart J 2018. [Epub ahead of print].

10. Dattilo P, Prasad A, Honeycutt E, et al. Contemporary patterns of fractional flow reserve and intravascular ultrasound use among patients undergoing percutaneous coronary intervention in the United States. J Am Coll Cardiol 2012;60(22):2337–9.

11. Sen S, Escaned J, Malik I, et al. Development and validation of a new adenosine-independent index of stenosis severity from coronary wave–intensity analysis. J Am Coll Cardiol 2012;59(15):1392–402.

12. Sen S, Asrress K, Nijjer S, et al. Diagnostic classification of the instantaneous wave-free ratio is

equivalent to fractional flow reserve and is not improved with adenosine administration. J Am Coll Cardiol 2013;61(13):1409–20.

13. Jeremias A, Maehara A, Généreux P, et al. Multicenter core laboratory comparison of the instantaneous wave-free ratio and resting P d/P a with fractional flow reserve. J Am Coll Cardiol 2014; 63(13):1253–61.

14. Escaned J, Echavarría-Pinto M, Garcia-Garcia H, et al. Prospective assessment of the diagnostic accuracy of instantaneous wave-free ratio to assess coronary stenosis relevance. JACC Cardiovasc Interv 2015;8(6):824–33.

15. Petraco R, Al-Lamee R, Gotberg M, et al. Real-time use of instantaneous wave–free ratio: Results of the ADVISE in-practice: an international, multicenter evaluation of instantaneous wave–free ratio in clinical practice. Am Heart J 2014;168(5):739–48.

16. Maini R, Moscona J, Katigbak P, et al. Instantaneous wave-free ratio as an alternative to fractional flow reserve in assessment of moderate coronary stenoses: a meta-analysis of diagnostic accuracy studies. Cardiovasc Revasc Med 2018;19(5):613–20.

17. Berry C, van 't Veer M, Witt N, et al. VERIFY (VERification of instantaneous wave-free ratio and fractional flow reserve for the assessment of coronary artery stenosis severity in everyday practice). J Am Coll Cardiol 2013;61(13):1421–7.

18. Hennigan B, Oldroyd K, Berry C, et al. Discordance between resting and hyperemic indices of coronary stenosis severity. Circ Cardiovasc Interv 2016;9(11): e004016.

19. Davies J, Sen S, Dehbi H, et al. Use of the instantaneous wave-free ratio or fractional flow reserve in PCI. N Engl J Med 2017;376(19):1824–34.

20. Götberg M, Christiansen E, Gudmundsdottir I, et al. Instantaneous wave-free ratio versus fractional flow reserve to guide PCI. N Engl J Med 2017;376(19):1813–23.

21. Barbato E, Toth G, Johnson N, et al. A prospective natural history study of coronary atherosclerosis using fractional flow reserve. J Am Coll Cardiol 2016; 68(21):2247–55.

22. Escaned J, Ryan N, Mejía-Rentería H, et al. Safety of the deferral of coronary revascularization on the basis of instantaneous wave-free ratio and fractional flow reserve measurements in stable coronary artery disease and acute coronary syndromes. JACC Cardiovasc Interv 2018;11(15): 1437–49.

23. Berry C, McClure J, Oldroyd K. Meta-analysis of death and myocardial infarction in the DEFINE-FLAIR and iFR-SWEDEHEART trials. Circulation 2017;136(24):2389–91.

24. Lee J, Shin E, Nam C, et al. Clinical outcomes according to fractional flow reserve or instantaneous wave-free ratio in deferred lesions. JACC Cardiovasc Interv 2017;10(24):2502–10.

25. Escaned J, Collet C, Ryan N, et al. Clinical outcomes of state-of-the-art percutaneous coronary revascularization in patients with de novo three vessel disease: 1-year results of the SYNTAX II study. Eur Heart J 2017;38(42):3124–34.

26. Van Belle E, Gil R, Klauss V, et al. Impact of routine invasive physiology at time of angiography in patients with multivessel coronary artery disease on reclassification of revascularization strategy. JACC Cardiovasc Interv 2018;11(4): 354–65.

27. Kikuta Y, Cook C, Sharp A, et al. Pre-angioplasty instantaneous wave-free ratio pullback predicts hemodynamic outcome in humans with coronary artery disease. JACC Cardiovasc Interv 2018;11(8): 757–67.

28. Kobayashi Y, Johnson N, Berry C, et al. The influence of lesion location on the diagnostic accuracy of adenosine-free coronary pressure wire measurements. JACC Cardiovasc Interv 2016;9(23):2390–9.

Technical Approaches to Left Main Coronary Intervention
Contemporary Best Practices

Tanveer Rab, MD, FSCAI

KEYWORDS

• Left main coronary intervention • Percutaneous techniques

KEY POINTS

• In Left Main stenosis, distal left main bifurcation lesion is most common. Technical approaches are driven by lesion complexity in the ostial/proximal left circumflex side branch.
• A single-stent strategy using provisional stenting should be used for simple lesions involving the distal left main bifurcation, with a crossover to a two stent technique, if the left circumflex side branch is compromised.
• A 2-stent strategy should be used for complex lesions of the distal left main; the double kiss (DK) Crush technique may provides the most optimal results compared with other strategies.
• Postprocedure intravascular imaging is strongly recommended as it is associated with improved outcomes after left main stenting.

INTRODUCTION

Left main (LM) percutaneous coronary intervention (PCI) is an acceptable alternative to coronary artery bypass grafting (CABG), and in experienced hands, excellent procedural results can be obtained. A systematic approach to stenting and meticulous attention to detail are required. For most lesions, a single-stent provisional approach is sufficient, but for the more complex lesion, a 2-stent technique is required. The goals of LM stenting are to safely perform the PCI procedure[1] to reduce immediate procedural complications and reduce long-term target vessel failure, which may require target lesion revascularization.[2–4]

INDICATIONS FOR LEFT MAIN PERCUTANEOUS CORONARY INTERVENTION

A combination of angiographic and imaging criteria is used to guide the decision to intervene on the LM.[2] These criteria include the severity of stenosis, as defined by angiography, intravascular imaging, and physiologic assessment. Standard criteria for intervention include an angiographic stenosis greater than 70%,[5,6] a minimal luminal area (MLA) ≤ 6 mm^2,[7] and fractional flow reserve (FFR) of ≤ 0.80 in the setting of lesions that are of intermediate angiographic severity ($>50\%$ to $<90\%$).[8,9] (Box 1)

LESION CHARACTERISTICS AND IMPACT ON APPROACH TO LEFT MAIN PERCUTANEOUS CORONARY INTERVENTION
Lesion Complexity

LM stenosis is seen in 5% to 7% of coronary angiograms.[10–12] As many as 80% of these stenoses involve the left main bifurcation (LMB).[5,6] Stenting strategies are driven by the extent of disease involving the side branch (SB). To stratify the best LM stenting strategy, LMB are classified as *simple* or *complex* (Fig. 1), based on the

---

Interventional Cardiology, Emory University School of Medicine, 1364 Clifton road, NE, Suite F 606, Atlanta, GA 30322, USA
E-mail address: srab@emory.edu
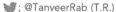 ; @TanveerRab (T.R.)

Intervent Cardiol Clin 8 (2019) 131–147
https://doi.org/10.1016/j.iccl.2018.11.004
2211-7458/19/© 2018 Elsevier Inc. All rights reserved.

Box 1
Criteria for left main intervention

- Angiographic stenosis greater than 70%
- Intravascular ultrasound (IVUS) or optical coherence tomography (OCT) minimal luminal area (MLA) ≤ 6 mm^2
- Fractional flow reserve (FFR) of ≤ 0.80 (with intermediate lesions >50% to <90%)
---

criteria in the Definitions and impact of complEx biFurcation lesIons on clinical outcomes after percutaNeous coronary IntervenTIOn using drug-eluting steNts (DEFINITION) study.[13] A *simple* LMB is a lesion with SB diameter stenosis less than 70% and a SB lesion length less than 10 mm. This is seen in 75% of cases and can be treated with a single-stent provisional approach. A *complex* LMB lesion has an SB stenosis greater than 70% and a SB lesion length greater than 10 mm. A simple lesion can change to a complex lesion with the presence of 2 of 6 minor criteria,[13] which involve the degree of calcification, bifurcation angle, reference vessel diameter, presence of thrombus, and main vessel lesion length (Box 2). Complex lesions generally require a 2-stent strategy.

Medina Classification

The Medina classification[14–16] is an angiographic classification of bifurcation lesion complexity that assists in defining plaque distribution and procedural planning but does not predict outcomes of PCI. The first numeral reflects the presence or absence of narrowing in the proximal main vessel (1 = present, 0 = absent); the second numeral reflects the presence or absence of narrowing in the distal main vessel, and the third numeral reflects the presence or absence of narrowing in the SB ostium. Medina class 1.1.1, 1.0.1, and 0.1.1 are true bifurcation lesions. The validity of this classification requires bifurcation-dedicated quantitative coronary angiography software.

Imaging and Functional Assessment

The size, angle, calcification, and length of the LM and daughter branches are assessed by intravascular ultrasound (IVUS) or optical coherence tomography (OCT) and its functional significance by FFR in both daughter branches (left anterior descending [LAD] and left circumflex [LCX]). Imaging by intravascular ultrasound (IVUS) or OCT can visualize plaque distribution, tissue characterization, arc of

calcification (270°–360°), and severity of stenosis (MLA ≤ 6 mm^2). IVUS MLA less than 5.9 mm^2 and an FFR of ≤ 0.80 are thresholds for intervention.[8] A limitation of OCT imaging in the LM is the image interference with blood in a field that should be bloodless and filled only with contrast, and therefore the inability to image the LM ostium. Power injection of 20 cc of contrast over 5 seconds, and a psi of 500 can improve image quality[17]

Anatomic and Clinical Complexity

Synergy Between Percutaneous Coronary Intervention With TAXUS and Cardiac Surgery (SYNTAX),[18] SYNTAX II,[19] NERS (New Risk Stratification) II,[20] and EuroScore (European System for Cardiac Operative Risk Evaluation)[21] are the most widely used scores to describe anatomic and clinical complexity. The Global Risk score combines SYNTAX with EuroSCORE to provide an algorithm to identify low-risk patients who can benefit from CABG or PCI.[22] The DEFINITION Study[13] criteria are the only specific risk score for LMB. The SYNTAX score had prior validation[23–27] in providing differential outcomes with PCI and CABG. However, in both the EXCEL (Everolimus-Eluting Stents or Bypass Surgery for Left Main Coronary Artery Disease) and the NOBLE (Nordic-Baltic-British left main revascularization) randomized trials of LM PCI compared with CABG, the SYNTAX score failed to clearly discriminate such outcomes, which partially might be attributed to different endpoints (and different drug-eluting stents) used in each trial. In a recent meta-analysis, cardiac mortality at a follow-up at 39 months was lower with PCI in patients with low SYNTAX score but increased with high SYNTAX score.[28]

Bifurcation Angle

The bifurcation angle can only be measured accurately with computed tomographic angiography. A wide angle between LM and the LAD artery is associated with a reduced event rate after stenting, because of lower target lesion revascularization (TLR).[29] The commonly referenced "bifurcation angle" (or angle B)[3] between the LAD and the LCX (70°-80°) did not predict clinical outcomes in the SYNTAX trial.[30] A wide LAD-LCX angle pre-PCI has been identified as a predictor of worse outcomes after Culotte and the classic Crush techniques.[31–33] However, in the DK-CRUSH III study (Randomized Study on Double Kissing Crush Technique Versus Provisional Stenting Technique for Coronary Artery Bifurcation Lesions)- double kissing (DK) Crush was associated with lower rates of major adverse

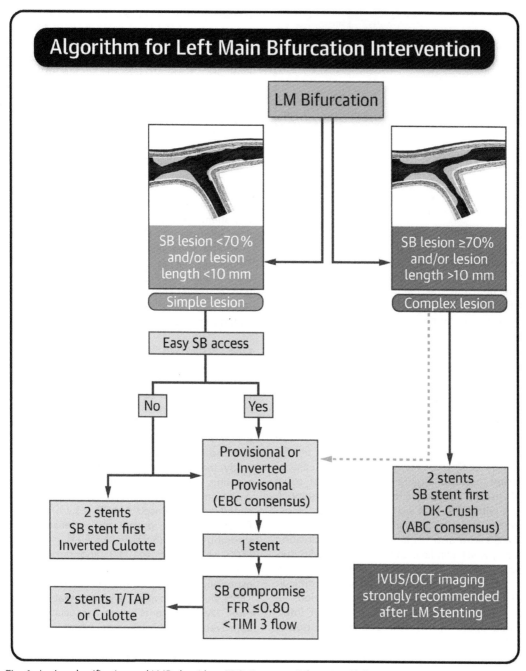

Fig. 1. Lesion classification and LMB algorithm. EBC, European Bifurcation Club; T, T stenting; TAP, T And Protrusion; TIMI, Thrombolysis in myocardial infarction. (*Adapted from* Rab T, Sheiban I, Louvard Y, et al. Current interventions for the left main bifurcation. JACC Cardiovasc Interv 2017;10(9):853; with permission.)

cardiovascular events (MACE) for the LMB compared with the Culotte technique when the bifurcation angle between the LAD and LCX was greater than 70°.[34] Therefore, for wider bifurcation angles or when the LCX is smaller than the LAD (but larger than 2 mm in diameter), DK Crush is the ideal 2-stent technique. If the bifurcation angle is less than 70° and the LCX

diameter is within 0.5 mm of the LAD diameter, either Culotte or DK Crush techniques can be performed.[35,36]

INTERVENTIONAL APPROACH
Access and Guiding Catheters
LM PCI can be performed by either the femoral or the radial approach. Stenting techniques can

> **Box 2**
> **Complex bifurcation lesions: minor criteria**
>
> - Moderate to severe calcification
> - Multiple lesions
> - Bifurcation angle >70°
> - Main vessel reference vessel diameter <2.5 mm
> - Thrombus containing lesion
> - Main vessel lesion length >25 mm
>
> Note. If 2 or more of minor criteria are present, an otherwise simple lesion (SB diameter stenosis <70% and lesion length <10 mm) is redefined as complex.

be performed with 6-French Extra Back Up 3.5/3.75 or Judkins JL 3.5/4 guiding catheters (with side holes) if the LM ostium is diseased. A 7-French or 8-French guide catheter can be used for large-caliber coronaries, rotational atherectomy (RA) burr sizes ≥1.75 mm, or rarely, if 2 stents must be delivered simultaneously.

Main Branch and Side Branch Wiring

Both branches of the LMB should be wired with the most difficult branch wired first. The second wire is then inserted while limiting rotation to avoid wrap with the first wire. Wiring the SB (ie, the LCX) provides a safety net in case of abrupt occlusion, generally in cases of ostial SB disease of greater than 50% in severity. A wire within the LCX also facilitates flow recovery by acting as a marker for SB rewiring.[37] The SB wire also helps change the bifurcation angle, which can facilitate access to the SB during guidewire exchange. Deflectable and angulated microcatheters can assist in difficult SB wiring.[3] In the author's opinion, a SB <2.0 mm should be wired but not intervened upon. Microscopic evaluation suggests that polymer-coated wires, when jailed, are more resistant to retrieval damage and were more efficient in crossing the SB ostium than non–polymer-coated wires.[38]

Optimal Lesion Preparation and the Calcified Vessel

Noncompliant and scoring balloons are used to optimize lesion preparation for stent delivery. RA is required for the nondilatable or severely calcified LM lesion. In the PROTECT II trial, which randomly assigned patients undergoing nonemergent, high-risk PCI to either Impella (Abiomed, Danvers, MA, USA) or intra-aortic balloon pump (IABP), RA was used in 8% of cases in the Impella arm compared with 3.1% in the IABP arm. RA averaged 5 passes, with total RA time of 60 seconds in the Impella arm compared with 40 seconds in the IABP arm and was associated with increased rates of myocardial infarction (MI) (13.8% vs 10.4%). Adverse events can be reduced with short-duration RA at a speed between 140,000 and 180,000 rpm with less than 3 passes and burr advances of less than 10 seconds, using burr sizes of 1.5 mm and 1.75 mm.[39] Caution should be exercised in angulated lesions where wire bias can cause vessel perforation. In a small series of patients in whom RA was performed in calcified unprotected left main (UPLM) stenosis, TLR rates were less than 20% at 2 years.[39,40] Temporary pacing is recommended when RA is used in high-risk PCI with low ejection fraction (EF). A smaller series of patients have safely undergone orbital atherectomy of the calcified LM with no adverse safety concerns.[41,42]

One versus Two Stents

There is a lack of randomized studies comparing 1- versus 2-stent techniques for LMB. The COBIS (Coronary Bifurcation Stenting) II registry[43] reported a higher incidence of cardiac death, MI, and target lesion failure after 2 stents for LMB. The DKCRUSH-III study[34,35] was the only randomized, multicenter, 2-stent study that compared DK Crush with Culotte stenting for patients with distal LMB lesions. At 3-year follow-up, Culotte stenting was associated with increased MACE (23.7% vs 8.2%, P<.001), mainly driven by increased stent thrombosis (ST) (3.9% vs 0.5%, P = .02), MI (8.2% vs 3.4%, P = .037), and target vessel revascularization (18.8% vs 5.8%, P<.001), especially in complex LMB lesion. The DEFINITION study[13] provided evidence that for complex LM, 2 stents were associated with improved clinical outcomes when compared with a 1-stent strategy.

DK Crush stenting technique[44] is a modification of the classic Crush technique. Following the results of DK CRUSH-V study,[45] which compared DK Crush stenting versus provisional stenting (PS) (1-year target lesion failure of 4.8% vs 18%), a 2-stent DK Crush technique is the procedure of choice for the complex LMB lesion. The ongoing European Bifurcation Club Left Main (NCT02497014)[46] is a randomized trial comparing 1 versus 2 stents for the LMB and may further provide important information regarding the optimal treatment of LMB bifurcation lesions.

Stenting Techniques Based on Lesion Location

Ostial and midshaft stenoses are simple lesions. An MLA by IVUS of $\leq$4.5 mm^2 is an added criterion for functional significance and correlates with an FFR of $\leq$0.80.[47] Stenting lesions at these locations with drug-eluting stents (DES) is associated with better clinical outcomes than stenting at the LMB. In the Delta registry, the rates of MACE at 3-year follow-up for these simple lesions were 19.1% versus 28.5%; target vessel revascularization, 9.3% versus 17.7%; and target lesion revascularization, 4.5% versus 12.6%.[48] In the setting of a long LM, an 8-mm or 12-mm stent may provide adequate coverage for an ostial or shaft lesion. Left anterior oblique (LAO) caudal and cranial views should be used for stent positioning. **Fig. 2** demonstrates stent positioning in the LAO cranial view with a second wire in the cusp acting as the "marker wire." The crossing point of the coronary and marker wires suggests the ostium of the LM and a 1- to 2-mm protrusion of the stent into the cusp ensures adequate ostial coverage. A short LM with ostial stenosis should be treated with the provisional technique (described in later discussion), as the distal portion of the stent will extend beyond the LMB.

For lesions involving the LMB, expertise in 4 stenting techniques is recommended: PS (**Fig. 3**); T and minimal protrusion (TAP) (**Fig. 4**); Culotte (**Fig. 5**); and DK Crush (**Fig. 6**). An algorithm for LMB intervention recommends stenting strategies based on lesion complexity (see **Fig. 1**).

PROVISIONAL STENTING

A single-stent strategy using PS should be used for simple LMB lesions (see **Fig. 3**). Randomized studies suggest that the provisional SB stenting strategy is superior to a dedicated 2-stent approach and should be the recommended strategy.[49,50] In a subgroup of the SYNTAX trial, there was a lower rate of cardiac death at 5 years [51] and a lower 1-year MACE rate[30] with a PS approach. A 10-year follow-up of a large-propensity matched group of patients showed that patients treated with PS of the LMB had comparable rates of TLR compared with a 2-stent strategy.[52] Meta-analysis of 7 observational studies using DES for LM stenting demonstrated that compared with a 2-stent approach, a single-stent approach was associated with decreased rates of MACE (20.4% vs 32.8%) (odds ratio [OR], 0.51; 95% confidence interval [CI], 0.35–0.73) and target vessel revascularization (10.1% vs 24.3%) (OR, 0.35; 95% CI, 0.25–0.49).[53]

PS with a single-stent crossover from the LM into the LAD is the most common strategy in 75% of LMB interventions.[5,6] A 1-stent approach is favored in LMB lesions with nonsignificant ostial LCX stenosis of less than 50% with a lesion length of less than 5 mm, a non–left dominant coronary system, or an LCX less than 2.0 mm in diameter. If the predominant lesion is in the LCX and the ostium of the LAD is not diseased, a provisional 1-stent approach can be directed from the LM toward the LCX (also referred to as an inverted provisional approach).

Optimal visualization of the LMB and the SB ostium is achieved in LAO caudal ("spider" view) and AP (anteroposterior) or right anterior oblique caudal projections. The diameter of the LM stent must be carefully sized according to the diameter of the distal vessel (ie, the LAD). If an oversized stent is selected, it will increase not only the risk of distal dissection but also the risk of carinal shifting, which may result in

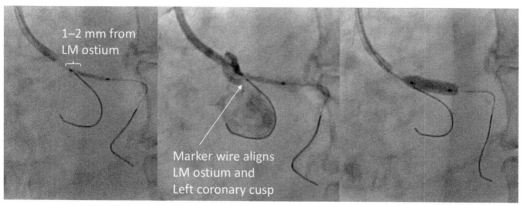

Fig. 2. Positioning ostial LM stent.

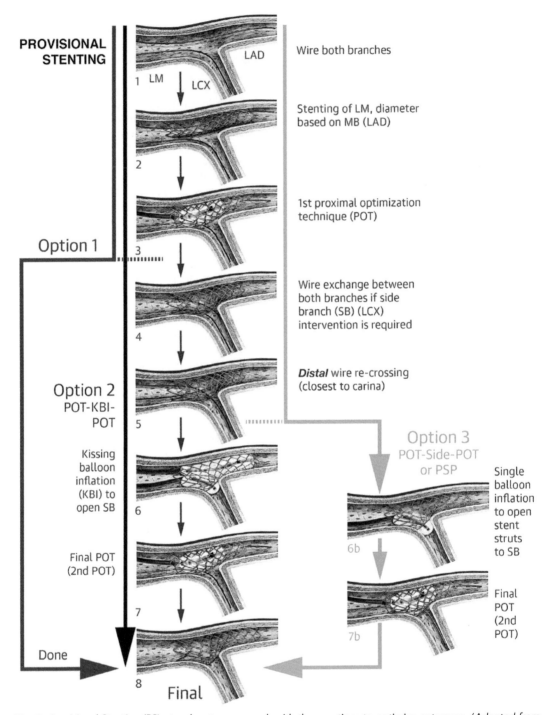

Fig. 3. Provisional Stenting (PS): step-by-step approach with three options to optimize outcomes. (*Adapted from* Rab T, Sheiban I, Louvard Y, et al. Current interventions for the left main bifurcation. JACC Cardiovasc Interv 2017;10(9):855; with permission.)

SB occlusion. Proximal optimization technique (POT) is then performed (described in later discussion). This allows strut protrusion into the SB with larger strut opening as well as no or limited carinal shifting for easier guidewire exchange.

Options for the Side Branch after Left Main Stent Implantation
After provisionally stenting the LMB, there are 3 options for the SB. For the simple lesion, crossover stenting followed by POT with no SB

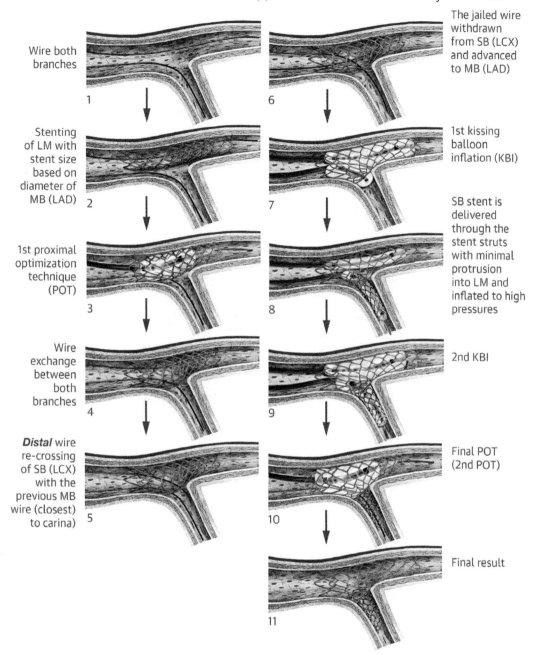

Wire both branches — 1

The jailed wire withdrawn from SB (LCX) and advanced to MB (LAD) — 6

Stenting of LM with stent size based on diameter of MB (LAD) — 2

1st kissing balloon inflation (KBI) — 7

1st proximal optimization technique (POT) — 3

SB stent is delivered through the stent struts with minimal protrusion into LM and inflated to high pressures — 8

Wire exchange between both branches — 4

2nd KBI — 9

Distal wire re-crossing of SB (LCX) with the previous MB wire (closest) to carina) — 5

Final POT (2nd POT) — 10

Final result — 11

Fig. 4. TAP technique: step-by-step approach. (*Adapted from* Rab T, Sheiban I, Louvard Y, et al. Current interventions for the left main bifurcation. JACC Cardiovasc Interv 2017;10(9):856; with permission.)

dilatation or kissing balloon inflations (KBI) is recommended. If intervention is required to the SB, guidewire exchange occurs. The main branch (MB) wire is pulled back and inserted into the SB through the most *distal cell* (closest to the carina), thus allowing the projection of struts in the ostial segment of the SB opposite the carina. The jailed SB wire is then pulled back and placed in the MB. An alternate technique using a fresh wire is to create a gentle double curve at the

tip, crossing the LM into the LAD with the tip pointing upwards and then gently pulling back with tip rotation downwards to enter the SB. POT, KBI, and re-POT are then performed. An alternate option (with no KBI) is POT-SB inflation and re-POT or PSP.[54,55] This optimizes the result of PS, maintaining circular geometry, reducing SB ostium strut obstruction and access to the LCX, risk of SB occlusion, and global strut malapposition. If the result of the SB is inadequate

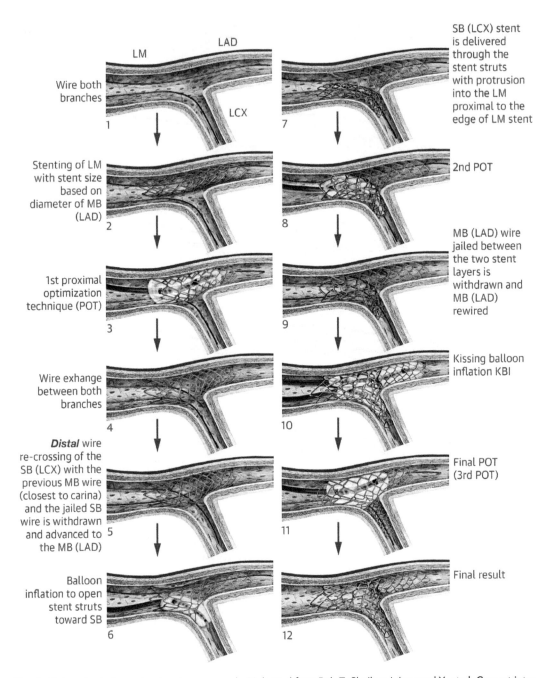

Fig. 5. Culotte technique: step-by-step approach. (*Adapted from* Rab T, Sheiban I, Louvard Y, et al. Current interventions for the left main bifurcation. JACC Cardiovasc Interv 2017;10(9):859; with permission.)

after MB stenting (Thrombolysis in Myocardial Infarction [TIMI] flow <III or an FFR of <0.75),[56] a second stent can be placed by the T, TAP, or Culotte techniques[57] after guidewire exchange.

Special care should be taken during LM stenting to avoid longitudinal stent compression, particularly with thin strut stents. Pullback of the jailed wire or a partially deflated balloon may deep seat the guiding catheter and damage

the stent. Optimal control of the guide with the left hand is thus crucial to avoid this complication (Fig. 7).

Proximal Optimization Technique

POT provides the LM crossover stent 2 distinct diameters corresponding to the diameters of the 2 covered segments (LAD and LM) that were derived by Murray's law (Fig. 8).[58] This

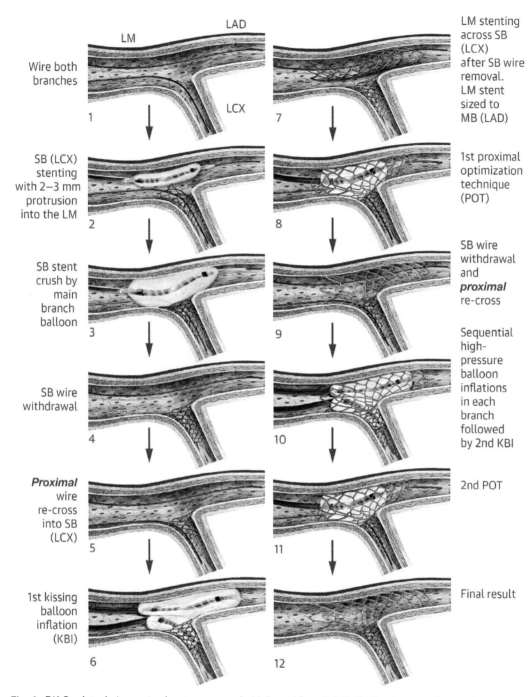

Fig. 6. DK Crush technique: step-by-step approach. (*Adapted from* Rab T, Sheiban I, Louvard Y, et al. Current interventions for the left main bifurcation. JACC Cardiovasc Interv 2017;10(9):865; with permission.)

technique allows the reconstruction of the initial physiologic anatomy of the bifurcation and follows the fractal law of Finet[59] whereby the LM final stent diameter = (Diameter of LAD + Diameter of LCX) × 0.67. POT facilitates wire exchange when SB treatment is needed by avoiding abluminal wire exchange outside the proximal part of the stent.[60] The stent should be implanted sufficiently proximal to the SB to accommodate a short, large-diameter balloon sized to the LM and at least 6 or 8 mm in length. Large-diameter (4.5 mm and 5.0 mm) stents are

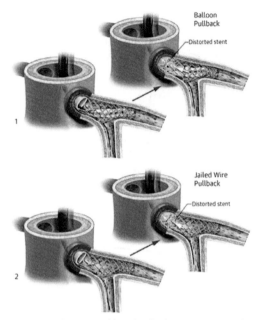

Fig. 7. Mechanisms of longitudinal stent compression and deformation in the LM. (*Adapted from* Rab T, Sheiban I, Louvard Y, et al. Current interventions for the left main bifurcation. JACC Cardiovasc Interv 2017;10(9):858; with permission.)

now commercially available. **Table 1** illustrates the expansion profiles of different stent types to accommodate the large LM caliber.[61] The distal marker of the POT balloon must be positioned in front of the carina (see **Fig. 8**). Optimization of the proximal stent segment allows strut protrusion with opening of cells toward the SB as well as no or limited carinal shifting for easier guidewire exchange, optimization of the stent diameter to the LM diameter, correcting malapposition, and reducing oval distortion of the stented segment after SB inflation or KBI.[55]

Kissing Balloon Inflations in Provisional Stenting
Routine KBI in the MB and SB after PS has failed to provide clear clinical benefits.[62–67] The 2-year

rate of the composite of death, MI, or TLR was not significantly different between KBI or no KBI, regardless of angiographic SB stenosis (12.5% in the final kissing balloon (FKB) group and 8.5% in the non-FKB group). Five-year follow-up of the DK CRUSH II study demonstrated that in the PS group, TLR with final KBI was 19.4% versus 5.2% without final KBI ($P = .31$).[68]

When necessary and to prevent potentially negative effects of KBI[63–66,69] (after rewiring the LCX through the distal portion of the cell overlying the SB), short noncompliant balloons are used in the unstented SB to prevent the occurrence of dissection and to avoid oval distortion in the LM. Balloon diameters are chosen according to Murray's law, and balloon inflation occurs in the SB first with simultaneous deflation of both balloons. To reduce proximal stent deformation when relatively long balloons are used, a "modified KBI approach" was recently proposed[54,62] using asymmetric inflation pressures: the SB is first inflated to 12 atm and then partly deflated back to 4 atm, with subsequent simultaneous inflation of both balloons at 12 atm with simultaneous deflation. Routine KBI is not recommended for a single-stent strategy, but a final KBI is mandatory in 2-stent techniques, including the PS strategy that converts to a 2-stent technique.

Crossover to a Two-Stent Strategy Using T-Stenting or T-And small-Protrusion
T-stenting or T-And small-Protrusion (TAP) (see **Fig. 4**) is used to optimize the SB in the setting of PS when a 1-stent approach was initially planned. Operators increasingly perform it as their go-to technique when an elective double-stenting strategy is required.[70] The LM stent is sized to the distal vessel, and after implantation, POT is performed. The jailed SB wire is withdrawn, and the SB is recrossed through a *distal* cell (closest to the carina). SB

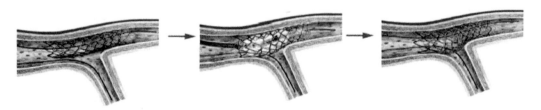

POT balloon should be 6–8 mm in length and sized to the LM with distal tip marker of the balloon position at the carina

Fig. 8. POT (proximal optimization technique).

Table 1
Stent expansion chart

Stent Type	Synergy	Resolute Integrity	Onyx	Onyx XL	Xience Alpine	Orsiro	Ultimaster	Biomatrix
Device company	Boston Scientific	Medtronic	Medtronic	Medtronic	Abbott Vascular	Biotronik	Terumo	Biosensors
Largest stent size (mm)	4.0	4.0	4.0	4.5–5.0	4.0	4.0	4.0	4.0
Crowns	10	9.5	9.5	10.5	9	6	8	9
Point connectors	2–5	3	2.5	2.5	3	3	2	3
Cell opening for SB access (mm)	1.09	1.03	1.03	1.03	1.11	1.04	0.99	1.37
Maximum stent expansion (mm), manufacturer's recommendation	5.7	4.75	4.75	5.75	4.6	4.4	4.57	4.5
Average stent expansion (mm), bench testing[77]	5.7	5.6	5.6	6.0	5.6	5.3	5.8	5.9

Adapted from Rab T, Sheiban I, Louvard Y, et al. Current interventions for the left main bifurcation. JACC Cardiovasc Interv 2017;10(9):849–65; with permission.

strut is dilated, and a second stent is implanted in the SB with minimal protrusion in the LM. An anticipated pitfall of this technique is that a single-layer "neocarina" is created by the SB stent struts protruding inside the LM at the level of the carina. The SB takeoff angle and site of strut crossing are major determinants of neocarina length. When the SB has a "T"-shape takeoff, a small amount of SB stent protrusion inside the LM is needed to cover the SB ostium successfully. On the other hand, acute SB angles (Y shapes) are associated with longer, oval-shaped SB ostia, which implies the need for wider protrusion of the SB stent inside the LM, resulting in a longer neocarina. For such reasons, striving to limit protrusion while implanting the SB stent is critical. KBI is the final step of the TAP technique. Deflations should be simultaneous; otherwise, the protruded stent in the LM will keep the same position as before KBI. In a recent study of 57 de novo LMB lesions treated with TAP stenting using second-generation DES had an acceptable target lesion failure (TLF) rate at 3-year follow-up of 13.3%.[71] In contrast, in the Bifurcations Bad Krozingen (BBK) II study, whereby 39% of patients underwent LM stenting, the Culotte technique had a numerically lower rate of TLF at 1 year compared with TAP had at 1 year (6.7% vs 12.0% [P = .11]).[72]

Crossover to a Two-Stent Strategy Using the Culotte Technique

The original Culotte stenting[57] with bare-metal stent (BMS) had been largely abandoned because of high restenosis rates. Since the introduction of DES, Culotte stenting has regained its popularity. In the setting of crossover after PS (LM to LAD), the approach is termed an inverted Culotte, which is the same technique as a standard Culotte but with the second stent extending from the LM into the SB (see **Fig. 5**). In an in vitro study of Culotte stenting,[73] proximal SB recrossing as opposed to distal SB recrossing resulted in more unopposed struts at the ostium, a neostent carina formation, and reduction of the struts-free SB ostial area. Stent underexpansion is recognized as an independent predictor of ST and restenosis with restriction of stent expansion like a "napkin ring" in Culotte stenting using closed-cell design stents.[62] However, even with open-cell design stents in the LMB, significant stent underexpansion in either the LM or the SB ostium was noted with Culotte stenting in contrast to DK Crush stenting.[34,35]

INTENTIONAL TWO-STENT TECHNIQUES
Double Kissing Crush Stenting

The DK Crush stenting technique is a modification of the classic Crush technique and has gained popularity as the preferred 2-stent LM technique for the complex lesion (see **Fig. 6**).[34,35,44] The importance of this technique was reflected in the most recent 2018 European Society of Cardiology (ESC) guidelines for myocardial revascularization where it recieved a Class IIb recommendation for true left main bifurcation lesions over provisional T stenting.[74] The main difference between classic and DK Crush is the use of first KBI. After balloon Crush of the implanted SB stent, which protrudes minimally into the LM, there are 2 layers of stent struts at the ostial SB. First, KBI optimizes the distorted SB stent, leaving only one layer of metal struts at the ostial SB, while minimizing repeated distortion of ostial SB stent with LM stent deployment, and facilitates the final KBI after LM stenting. Careful attention should be paid to rewiring the SB from the *proximal* stent cell as distal SB recrossing increases the possibility of the wire traversing the abluminal area between the stent and the vessel wall, leaving a significant gap at the SB ostium after final KBI. The methods to confirm the exact position of the SB wire are as follows: visual assessment from fluoroscopy (orthogonal projections to confirm SB rewiring from the proximal stent cell [away from the carina], or guidance with IVUS or OCT positioned in the LM). Key points in DK Crush technique are (1) proximal wire recrossing; (2) the use of 2 stents; (3) 2 KBIs; and (4) 2 POT inflations.

POSTPROCEDURE EVALUATION

Postprocedure intravascular imaging with IVUS or OCT is strongly recommended. IVUS pullback should be performed from both the LAD and the LCX into the LM. Imaging can identify stent underexpansion, stent malapposition, edge dissections, or significant residual disease that might go undetected with conventional angiography.[75,76] OCT provides exquisite detail of stent apposition, coverage, and proximal (in the case of DK Crush) or distal SB guidewire crossing (in TAP and Culotte techniques) before balloon inflations. Postprocedural assessment with intravascular imaging also appears to influence patient outcomes. At 3-year follow-up in patients receiving DES for LM disease, a mortality benefit was seen with IVUS guidance versus angiography guidance (4.7% vs 16.0%).[75] In a pooled analysis of 4 registries, there was 90%

survival free from cardiac death, MI, or TLR at 3 years when IVUS was used for LM stenting compared with 80.7% when IVUS was not used (*P* = .03).[77] Randomized trials have however failed to show a clinical benefit from IVUS use.[78,79] Optimal results are seen when there is restoration of fractal LM anatomy as derived from Finet's formula.[59]

IVUS-determined final stent areas have been associated with improved outcomes and may be used to guide LM intervention. A minimal stent area (MSA) of at least 8.2 mm^2 in the body of the LM, 7.2 mm^2 at the bifurcation ("polygon of confluence"), 6.3 mm^2 in the proximal LAD, and 5.0 mm^2 in the proximal LCX are associated with better outcomes ("5-6-7-8" rule).[80] IVUS was used in 80% of cases in the EXCEL randomized clinical trial and an LM MSA of greater than 12.5 mm^2 had the best outcomes.[5] An ostial LCX MSA of less than 4 mm^2 is associated with an increased thrombotic and restenosis risk.[76,80] Criteria for optimal stent implantation are also applicable to OCT, which is superior to angiography.[81] FFR can be used to assess SB hemodynamic compromise after PCI when a residual angiographic stenosis is seen after intervention.[56]

APPROACHES TO OTHER LEFT MAIN LESION ANATOMIES
Trifurcation Left Main
Trifurcations are encountered in 10% of cases[52,82] and pose particular technical challenges. In these cases, a single-stent strategy is recommended. If SBs have limited disease, "triple kissing" balloon inflations are associated with good results.[52] When significant SB disease is present, any 2-stent technique might be used according to the specific anatomy; a minor SB (eg, LCX or ramus) is generally identified and treated with a "keep-it-open" approach. Favorable early and long-term results have been reported, even in true trifurcation lesions that are at high risk of restenosis.[82,83]

Isolated Ostial Left Anterior Descending or Left Circumflex Disease (Medina Classification 0-0-1)
For isolated ostial LAD lesions, a single cross-over into the LM using a PS approach, followed by POT, is recommended. For isolated ostial LCX lesions, a 2-stent strategy demonstrated lower TLR (3.2 vs 12.0%, *P* = .07) and TLF (4.8 vs 12.0%, *P* = .16) than the 1-stent group.[84,85]

HEMODYNAMIC SUPPORT

The global catheter ventricular assist device (cVAD) registry of Impella utilization reported a 47% incidence of LM disease in patients with left ventricular ejection fraction (LVEF) less than 35%.[86] PROTECT II was the only trial of left ventricular support in high-risk PCI that included LM intervention. This trial compared the Impella 2.5 with an IABP in patients with an average LVEF of 24%.[87] In-hospital mortality in the intention-to-treat population was 7.6% in the Impella group compared with 5.9% in the IABP group, and 6.2% compared with 6.9% in the per-protocol population. The rate of major adverse events was not different for patients with IABP or Impella at 30 days. However, there was a trend toward decreased major adverse events at 90 days in the Impella group compared with IABP: 40.6% versus 49.3% (*P* = .066) in the intention-to-treat population and 40.0% versus 51.0% (*P* = .023) in the per-protocol population.

LM intervention with Impella support constituted 51% of cases in the USPELLA (US Impella) registry.[88] In this registry, the rates of in-hospital death and 30-day mortality were 3.4% and 4%, respectively. The MACE rate was 8% in elective cases with a 12-month survival of 88%. Similarly, in the Europella (European Impella) registry,[89] in hospital mortality was 9.1%, 30-day survival was 94.5%, and the MACE rate was 12.4%. These outcomes resulted in the 2015 Food and Drug administration approval of the Impella devices (2.5 and CP) for high-risk PCI.[90] The Impella device is currently recommended for high-risk LM patients with a depressed LVEF of less than 35%.

SUMMARY

A step-by-step approach to LM stenting is critical for optimal procedural outcomes. Lesions should be evaluated for complexity to determine whether PS or 2-stent technique is preferred. In most cases, a single-stent provisional approach is sufficient.

REFERENCES

1. Xu B, Redfors B, Yang Y, et al. Impact of operator experience and volume on outcomes after left main coronary artery percutaneous coronary intervention. JACC Cardiovasc Interv 2016;9(20): 2086–93.
2. Rab T, Sheiban I, Louvard Y, et al. Current interventions for the left main bifurcation. JACC Cardiovasc Interv 2017;10(9):849–65.
3. Burzotta F, Lassen JF, Banning AP, et al. Percutaneous coronary intervention in left main coronary

artery disease: the 13th consensus document from the European Bifurcation Club. EuroIntervention 2018;14(1):112–20.

4. Fajadet J, Capodanno D, Stone GW. Management of left main disease: an update. Eur Heart J 2018;ehy238.

5. Stone GW, Sabik JF, Serruys PW, et al. Everolimus-eluting stents or bypass surgery for left main coronary artery disease. N Engl J Med 2016;375(23): 2223–35.

6. Mäkikallio T, Holm NR, Lindsay M, et al. Percutaneous coronary angioplasty versus coronary artery bypass grafting in treatment of unprotected left main stenosis (NOBLE): a prospective, randomised, open-label, non-inferiority trial. Lancet 2016; 388(10061):2743–52.

7. de la Torre Hernandez JM, Hernandez Hernandez F, Alfonso F, et al. Prospective application of pre-defined intravascular ultrasound criteria for assessment of intermediate left main coronary artery lesions results from the multicenter LITRO study. J Am Coll Cardiol 2011;58(4):351–8.

8. Jasti V, Ivan E, Yalamanchili V, et al. Correlations between fractional flow reserve and intravascular ultrasound in patients with an ambiguous left main coronary artery stenosis. Circulation 2004; 110(18):2831–6.

9. Authors/Task Force members, Windecker S, Kolh P, Alfonso F, et al. 2014 ESC/EACTS Guidelines on myocardial revascularization: the task force on myocardial revascularization of the European Society of Cardiology (ESC) and the European Association for Cardio-Thoracic Surgery (EACTS) Developed with the special contribution of the European Association of Percutaneous Cardiovascular Interventions (EAPCI). Eur Heart J 2014;35(37): 2541–619.

10. De Caterina AR, Cuculi F, Banning AP. Incidence, predictors and management of left main coronary artery stent restenosis: a comprehensive review in the era of drug-eluting stents. EuroIntervention 2013;8(11):1326–34.

11. DeMots H, Rosch J, McAnulty JH, et al. Left main coronary artery disease. Cardiovasc Clin 1977;8(2): 201–11.

12. Taylor HA, Deumite NJ, Chaitman BR, et al. Asymptomatic left main coronary artery disease in the Coronary Artery Surgery Study (CASS) registry. Circulation 1989;79(6):1171–9.

13. Chen S-L, Sheiban I, Xu B, et al. Impact of the complexity of bifurcation lesions treated with drug-eluting StentsThe DEFINITION Study (Definitions and impact of complEx biFurcation lesIons on clinical outcomes after percutaNeous coronary IntervenTIOn using drug-eluting steNts). JACC Cardiovasc Interv 2014; 7(11):1266–76.

14. Medina A, Suarez de Lezo J, Pan M. A new classification of coronary bifurcation lesions. Rev Esp Cardiol 2006;59(2):183 [in Spanish].

15. Lassen JF, Holm NR, Banning AP, et al. Percutaneous coronary intervention for coronary bifurcation disease: 11th consensus document from the European Bifurcation Club. EuroIntervention 2016; 12(1):38–46.

16. Louvard Y, Thomas M, Dzavik V, et al. Classification of coronary artery bifurcation lesions and treatments: time for a consensus! Catheter Cardiovasc Interv 2008;71(2):175–83.

17. Bing R, Yong ASC, Lowe HC. Percutaneous transcatheter assessment of the left main coronary arterycurrent status and future directions. JACC Cardiovasc Interv 2015;8(12):1529–39.

18. Sianos G, Morel MA, Kappetein AP, et al. The SYNTAX Score: an angiographic tool grading the complexity of coronary artery disease. EuroIntervention 2005;1(2):219–27.

19. Farooq V, van Klaveren D, Steyerberg EW, et al. Anatomical and clinical characteristics to guide decision making between coronary artery bypass surgery and percutaneous coronary intervention for individual patients: development and validation of SYNTAX score II. Lancet 2013;381(9867): 639–50.

20. Chen SL, Han YL, Zhang YJ, et al. The anatomic-and clinical-based NERS (new risk stratification) score II to predict clinical outcomes after stenting unprotected left main coronary artery disease: results from a multicenter, prospective, registry study. JACC Cardiovasc Interv 2013;6(12):1233–41.

21. Gogbashian A, Sedrakyan A, Treasure T. EuroSCORE: a systematic review of international performance. Eur J Cardiothoracic Surg 2004;25(5):695–700.

22. Serruys PW, Farooq V, Vranckx P, et al. A global risk approach to identify patients with left main or 3-vessel disease who could safely and efficaciously be treated with percutaneous coronary interventionthe syntax trial at 3 years. JACC Cardiovasc Interv 2012;5(6):606–17.

23. Garg S, Stone GW, Kappetein A-P, et al. Clinical and angiographic risk assessment in patients with left main stem lesions. JACC Cardiovasc Interv 2010;3(9):891–901.

24. Tiroch K, Mehilli J, Byrne RA, et al. Impact of coronary anatomy and stenting technique on long-term outcome after drug-eluting stent implantation for unprotected left main coronary artery disease. JACC Cardiovasc Interv 2014;7(1):29–36.

25. Xhepa E, Tada T, Kufner S, et al. Long-term prognostic value of risk scores after drug-eluting stent implantation for unprotected left main coronary artery: a pooled analysis of the ISAR-LEFT-MAIN and ISAR-LEFT-MAIN 2 randomized clinical trials. Catheter Cardiovasc Interv 2017;89(1):1–10.

26. Morice M-C, Serruys PW, Kappetein AP, et al. Five-year outcomes in patients with left main disease treated with either percutaneous coronary intervention or coronary artery bypass grafting in the SYNTAX trial. Circulation 2014;129(23):2388–94.

27. Cavalcante R, Sotomi Y, Lee CW, et al. Outcomes after percutaneous coronary intervention or bypass surgery in patients with unprotected left main disease. J Am Coll Cardiol 2016;68(10):999–1009.

28. Palmerini T, Serruys P, Kappetein AP, et al. Clinical outcomes with percutaneous coronary revascularization vs coronary artery bypass grafting surgery in patients with unprotected left main coronary artery disease: a meta-analysis of 6 randomized trials and 4,686 patients. Am Heart J 2017;190:54–63.

29. Amemiya K, Domei T, Iwabuchi M, et al. Impact of the bifurcation angle on major cardiac events after cross-over single stent strategy in unprotected left main bifurcation lesions: 3-dimensional quantitative coronary angiographic analysis. Am J Cardiovasc Dis 2014;4(4):168–76.

30. Girasis C, Farooq V, Diletti R, et al. Impact of 3-dimensional bifurcation angle on 5-year outcome of patients after percutaneous coronary intervention for left main coronary artery disease: a substudy of the SYNTAX trial (synergy between percutaneous coronary intervention with taxus and cardiac surgery). JACC Cardiovasc Interv 2013;6(12):1250–60.

31. Adriaenssens T, Byrne RA, Dibra A, et al. Culotte stenting technique in coronary bifurcation disease: angiographic follow-up using dedicated quantitative coronary angiographic analysis and 12-month clinical outcomes. Eur Heart J 2008; 29(23):2868–76.

32. Dzavik V, Kharbanda R, Ivanov J, et al. Predictors of long-term outcome after crush stenting of coronary bifurcation lesions: importance of the bifurcation angle. Am Heart J 2006;152(4):762–9.

33. Song PS, Song YB, Lee JM, et al. Major predictors of long-term clinical outcomes after percutaneous coronary intervention for coronary bifurcation lesions with 2-stent strategypatient-level analysis of the Korean Bifurcation Pooled Cohorts. JACC Cardiovasc Interv 2016;9(18):1879–86.

34. Chen SL, Xu B, Han YL, et al. Comparison of double kissing crush versus Culotte stenting for unprotected distal left main bifurcation lesions: results from a multicenter, randomized, prospective DKCRUSH-III study. J Am Coll Cardiol 2013;61(14): 1482–8.

35. Chen SL, Xu B, Han YL, et al. Clinical outcome after DK crush versus culotte stenting of distal left main bifurcation lesions: the 3-year follow-up results of the DKCRUSH-III study. JACC Cardiovasc Interv 2015;8(10):1335–42.

36. Lefèvre T, Girasis C, Lassen JF. Differences between the left main and other bifurcations. EuroIntervention 2015;11(V):V106–10.

37. Hahn JY, Chun WJ, Kim JH, et al. Predictors and outcomes of side branch occlusion after main vessel stenting in coronary bifurcation lesions: results from the COBIS II registry (COronary BIfurcation Stenting). J Am Coll Cardiol 2013;62(18): 1654–9.

38. Pan M, Ojeda S, Villanueva E, et al. Structural damage of jailed guidewire during the treatment of coronary bifurcation lesions: a microscopic randomized trial. JACC Cardiovasc Interv 2016;9(18): 1917–24.

39. Garcia-Lara J, Pinar E, Valdesuso R, et al. Percutaneous coronary intervention with rotational atherectomy for severely calcified unprotected left main: immediate and two-years follow-up results. Catheter Cardiovasc Interv 2012;80(2):215–20.

40. Yabushita H, Takagi K, Tahara S, et al. Impact of rotational atherectomy on heavily calcified, unprotected left main disease. Circ J 2014;78(8):1867–72.

41. Lee MS, Shlofmitz E, Kong J, et al. Outcomes of patients with severely calcified aorto-ostial coronary lesions who underwent orbital atherectomy. J Interv Cardiol 2018;31(1):15–20.

42. Lee MS, Shlofmitz E, Shlofmitz R, et al. Outcomes after orbital atherectomy of severely calcified left main lesions: analysis of the ORBIT II study. J Invasive Cardiol 2016;28(9):364–9.

43. Song YB, Hahn J-Y, Yang JH, et al. Differential prognostic impact of treatment strategy among patients with left main versus non–left main bifurcation lesions undergoing percutaneous coronary interventionresults from the COBIS (Coronary Bifurcation Stenting) registry II. JACC Cardiovasc Interv 2014;7(3):255–63.

44. Zhang J-J, Chen S-L. Classic crush and DK crush stenting techniques. EuroIntervention 2015;11(V): V102–5.

45. Chen SL, Zhang JJ, Han Y, et al. Double kissing crush versus provisional stenting for left main distal bifurcation lesions: DKCRUSH-V randomized trial. J Am Coll Cardiol 2017;70(21):2605–17.

46. Chieffo A, Hildick-Smith D. The European Bifurcation Club Left Main Study (EBC MAIN): rationale and design of an international, multicentre, randomised comparison of two stent strategies for the treatment of left main coronary bifurcation disease. EuroIntervention 2016;12(1):47–52.

47. Park SJ, Ahn JM, Kang SJ, et al. Intravascular ultrasound-derived minimal lumen area criteria for functionally significant left main coronary artery stenosis. JACC Cardiovasc Interv 2014;7(8):868–74.

48. Naganuma T, Chieffo A, Meliga E, et al. Long-term clinical outcomes after percutaneous coronary intervention for ostial/mid-shaft lesions versus

distal bifurcation lesions in unprotected left main coronary artery: the DELTA Registry (drug-eluting stent for left main coronary artery disease): a multi-center registry evaluating percutaneous coronary intervention versus coronary artery bypass grafting for left main treatment. JACC Cardiovasc Interv 2013;6(12):1242–9.

49. D'Ascenzo F, Iannaccone M, Giordana F, et al. Provisional vs. two-stent technique for unprotected left main coronary artery disease after ten years follow up: a propensity matched analysis. Int J Cardiol 2016;211:37–42.

50. Palmerini T, Marzocchi A, Tamburino C, et al. Impact of bifurcation technique on 2-year clinical outcomes in 773 patients with distal unprotected left main coronary artery stenosis treated with drug-eluting stents. Circ Cardiovasc Interv 2008;1(3):185–92.

51. Toyofuku M, Kimura T, Morimoto T, et al. Comparison of 5-year outcomes in patients with and without unprotected left main coronary artery disease after treatment with sirolimus-eluting stents: insights from the j-Cypher registry. JACC Cardiovasc Interv 2013;6(7):654–63.

52. Kubo S, Kadota K, Sabbah M, et al. Clinical and angiographic outcomes after drug-eluting stent implantation with triple-kissing-balloon technique for left main trifurcation lesion: comparison of single-stent and multi-stent procedures. J Invasive Cardiol 2014;26(11):571–8.

53. Karrowni W, Makki N, Dhaliwal AS, et al. Single versus double stenting for unprotected left main coronary artery bifurcation lesions: a systematic review and meta-analysis. J Invasive Cardiol 2014; 26(6):229–33.

54. Foin N, Torii R, Mortier P, et al. Kissing balloon or sequential dilation of the side branch and main vessel for provisional stenting of bifurcations: lessons from micro-computed tomography and computational simulations. JACC Cardiovasc Interv 2012;5(1):47–56.

55. Finet G, Derimay F, Motreff P, et al. Comparative analysis of sequential proximal optimizing technique versus kissing balloon inflation technique in provisional bifurcation stenting: fractal coronary bifurcation bench test. JACC Cardiovasc Interv 2015;8(10):1308–17.

56. Koo BK, Kang HJ, Youn TJ, et al. Physiologic assessment of jailed side branch lesions using fractional flow reserve. J Am Coll Cardiol 2005;46(4): 633–7.

57. Chevalier B, Glatt B, Royer T, et al. Placement of coronary stents in bifurcation lesions by the "culotte" technique. Am J Cardiol 1998;82(8): 943–9.

58. Lefevre T, Darremont O, Albiero R. Provisional side branch stenting for the treatment of bifurcation lesions. EuroIntervention 2010;6(Suppl J):J65–71.

59. Finet G, Gilard M, Perrenot B, et al. Fractal geometry of arterial coronary bifurcations: a quantitative coronary angiography and intravascular ultrasound analysis. EuroIntervention 2008;3(4): 490–8. DOI410.

60. Darremont O, Leymarie JL, Lefevre T, et al. Technical aspects of the provisional side branch stenting strategy. EuroIntervention 2015;11(Suppl V): V86–90.

61. Ng J, Foin N, Ang HY, et al. Over-expansion capacity and stent design model: an update with contemporary DES platforms. Int J Cardiol 2016; 221:171–9.

62. Murasato Y, Finet G, Foin N. Final kissing balloon inflation: the whole story. EuroIntervention 2015; 11(Suppl V):V81–5.

63. Niemela M, Kervinen K, Erglis A, et al. Randomized comparison of final kissing balloon dilatation versus no final kissing balloon dilatation in patients with coronary bifurcation lesions treated with main vessel stenting: the Nordic-Baltic Bifurcation Study III. Circulation 2011;123(1):79–86.

64. Gwon HC, Hahn JY, Koo BK, et al. Final kissing ballooning and long-term clinical outcomes in coronary bifurcation lesions treated with 1-stent technique: results from the COBIS registry. Heart 2012;98(3):225–31.

65. Yu CW, Yang JH, Song YB, et al. Long-term clinical outcomes of final kissing ballooning in coronary bifurcation lesions treated with the 1-stent technique: results from the COBIS II registry (Korean Coronary Bifurcation Stenting Registry). JACC Cardiovasc Interv 2015;8(10):1297–307.

66. Song YB, Park TK, Hahn JY, et al. Optimal strategy for provisional side branch intervention in coronary bifurcation lesions: 3-year outcomes of the SMART-STRATEGY randomized trial. JACC Cardiovasc Interv 2016;9(6):517–26.

67. Park S-J, Ahn J-M, Park H-S, et al. TCT-234 is final kissing ballooning mandatory in the treatment of distal left main disease treated by simple cross over stenting? J Am Coll Cardiol 2014;64(11_S).

68. Chen S-L, Santoso T, Zhang J-J, et al. Clinical outcome of double kissing crush versus provisional stenting of coronary artery bifurcation lesions. The 5-year follow-up results from a randomized and multicenter DKCRUSH-II study (Randomized study on double kissing crush technique versus provisional stenting technique for coronary artery bifurcation lesions). Circ Cardiovasc Interv 2017;10(2) [pii:e004497].

69. Mylotte D, Routledge H, Harb T, et al. Provisional side branch-stenting for coronary bifurcation lesions: evidence of improving procedural and clinical outcomes with contemporary techniques. Catheter Cardiovasc Interv 2013;82(4): E437–45.

70. Burzotta F, Dzavik V, Ferenc M, et al. Technical aspects of the T and small protrusion (TAP) technique. EuroIntervention 2015;11(Suppl V): V91–5.

71. Jabbour RJ, Tanaka A, Pagnesi M, et al. T-stenting with small protrusion: the default strategy for bailout provisional stenting? JACC Cardiovasc Interv 2016;9(17):1853–4.

72. Ferenc M, Gick M, Comberg T, et al. Culotte stenting vs. TAP stenting for treatment of de-novo coronary bifurcation lesions with the need for side-branch stenting: the Bifurcations Bad Krozingen (BBK) II angiographic trial. Eur Heart J 2016; 37(45):3399–405.

73. Zhang JM, Gao X, Li M, et al. Two-stent techniques for coronary artery bifurcation stenting: insights from imaging of bench deployments. J Clin Innov Cardiol 2016;1:15–23.

74. Neuman FJ, Sousa UM, Alfonso F, et al. 2018 ESC/ EACTS Guidelines for myocardial revascularization. Eur Heart J 2018.

75. Park SJ, Kim YH, Park DW, et al. Impact of intravascular ultrasound guidance on long-term mortality in stenting for unprotected left main coronary artery stenosis. Circ Cardiovasc Interv 2009;2(3):167–77.

76. Kang SJ, Ahn JM, Song H, et al. Comprehensive intravascular ultrasound assessment of stent area and its impact on restenosis and adverse cardiac events in 403 patients with unprotected left main disease. Circ Cardiovasc Interv 2011;4(6):562–9.

77. de la Torre Hernandez JM, Baz Alonso JA, Gomez Hospital JA, et al. Clinical impact of intravascular ultrasound guidance in drug-eluting stent implantation for unprotected left main coronary disease: pooled analysis at the patient-level of 4 registries. JACC Cardiovasc Interv 2014;7(3):244–54.

78. Chieffo A, Latib A, Caussin C, et al. A prospective, randomized trial of intravascular-ultrasound guided compared to angiography guided stent implantation in complex coronary lesions: the AVIO trial. Am Heart J 2013;165(1):65–72.

79. Jakabcin J, Spacek R, Bystron M, et al. Long-term health outcome and mortality evaluation after invasive coronary treatment using drug eluting stents with or without the IVUS guidance. Randomized control trial. HOME DES IVUS. Catheter Cardiovasc Interv 2010;75(4):578–83.

80. Park S-J, Ahn J-M, Kang S-J. Unprotected left main percutaneous coronary intervention: integrated use of fractional flow reserve and intravascular ultrasound. J Am Heart Assoc 2012;1(6):e004556.

81. Parodi G, Maehara A, Giuliani G, et al. Optical coherence tomography in unprotected left main coronary artery stenting. EuroIntervention 2010; 6(1):94–9.

82. Ielasi A, Takagi K, Latib A, et al. Long-term clinical outcomes following drug-eluting stent implantation for unprotected distal trifurcation left main disease: the Milan-New Tokyo (MITO) registry. Catheter Cardiovasc Interv 2014;83(4): 530–8.

83. Sheiban I, Gerasimou A, Bollati M, et al. Early and long-term results of percutaneous coronary intervention for unprotected left main trifurcation disease. Catheter Cardiovasc Interv 2009;73(1): 25–31.

84. Jang WJ, Song YB, Hahn JY, et al. Impact of bifurcation stent technique on clinical outcomes in patients with a Medina 0,0,1 coronary bifurcation lesion: results from the COBIS (COronary BIfurcation Stenting) II registry. Catheter Cardiovasc Interv 2014;84(5):E43–50.

85. Lee HM, Nam CW, Cho YK, et al. Long-term outcomes of simple crossover stenting from the left main to the left anterior descending coronary artery. Korean J Intern Med 2014;29(5): 597–602.

86. Maini B, Moses J, Dixon S, et al. TCT-24 global cVAD registry: a global initiative in percutaneous circulatory support from the cVAD steering committee on behalf of all cVAD Investigators. J Am Coll Cardiol 2016;68(18_S):B10.

87. O'Neill WW, Kleiman NS, Moses J, et al. A prospective, randomized clinical trial of hemodynamic support with Impella 2.5 versus intraaortic balloon pump in patients undergoing high-risk percutaneous coronary intervention: the PROTECT II study. Circulation 2012;126(14):1717–27.

88. Maini B, Naidu SS, Mulukutla S, et al. Real-world use of the Impella 2.5 circulatory support system in complex high-risk percutaneous coronary intervention: the USpella Registry. Catheter Cardiovasc Interv 2012;80(5):717–25.

89. Sjauw KD, Konorza T, Erbel R, et al. Supported high-risk percutaneous coronary intervention with the Impella 2.5 device the Europella registry. J Am Coll Cardiol 2009;54(25):2430–4.

90. U.S. Food and Drug Administration. FDA approves blood pump system to help patients maintain stable heart function during certain high-risk cardiac procedures. Available at: https://www.fda.gov/ NewsEvents/Newsroom/PressAnnouncements/ ucm439529.htm. Accessed March 7, 2017.

Robotic-Assisted Percutaneous Coronary Intervention
Concept, Data, and Clinical Application

Daniel Walters, MD, Jad Omran, MD, Mitul Patel, MD*,
Ryan Reeves, MD, Lawrence Ang, MD,
Ehtisham Mahmud, MD

KEYWORDS

- Percutaneous coronary intervention • Robotics • Coronary artery disease • Radiation safety
- Interventional device innovation

KEY POINTS

- Percutaneous coronary interventions expose the operators to radiation and orthopedic hazards.
- Robotic technology has been developed and proven to be safe and effective to perform simple and complex percutaneous coronary interventions from a remote cockpit.
- The evolution of robotic technology has the potential to allow for percutaneous coronary interventions to be performed remotely over long distances.

INTRODUCTION

Since the advent of percutaneous coronary intervention (PCI) with the first balloon angioplasty performed by Gruntzig and colleagues[1] in 1977, there have been a multitude of advances in the field. The development of drug-eluting stents, improvements in periprocedural pharmacotherapy, and innovations in intracoronary technology, including atherectomy devices and guidewire enhancements, have led to worldwide adoption of PCI as the most commonly used method of treating symptomatic coronary artery disease. Despite decades of evolution, however, the fundamental components of the PCI procedure itself remain largely unchanged. One or more operators stand tableside and are exposed to significant radiation while manually performing the procedure and wearing heavy lead aprons, eye protection, and head garments enabling only partial protection from radiation exposure. An increased focus on occupational hazards posed to interventional cardiologists shows growing evidence of cataracts, malignancy, and orthopedic injury resulting from work within the radiation field.[2–5] Since 1985, robotic systems to remove the practitioner from tableside have been in use in the surgical arena and refinements have been made.[6] Robotic technology is now available in interventional cardiology with the introduction of platforms through which PCI can be performed. The original system, a remote navigation system called RNS (NaviCath, Haifa, Israel) was a table-mounted motorized drive connected to a joystick-controlled operator module.[7] This led to the development and eventual approval of the CorPath robotic system (Corindus Vascular

---

Disclosure Statement: E. Mahmud has received research support from Corindus Vascular Robotics. R. Reeves has received consulting honorarium from Corindus Vascular Robotics.
Division of Cardiovascular Medicine, Sulpizio Cardiovascular Center, University of California, San Diego, 9434 Medical Center Drive, La Jolla, CA 92037, USA
* Corresponding author. Sulpizio Cardiovascular Center, University of California, San Diego, 9452 Medical Center Drive #7411, La Jolla, CA, 92037.
E-mail address: mpatel@ucsd.edu

Robotics, Waltham, MA, USA) for robotic-assisted PCI (R-PCI). The system removes the operator from the tableside and has been validated for safety, feasibility, and long-term efficacy in simple and complex lesions.[8–10]

OCCUPATIONAL HAZARDS IN THE CARDIAC CATHETERIZATION LABORATORY

The evolution of interventional cardiology procedures over the past 4 decades has allowed for a new array of complex procedures. These include a new era of technically difficult interventions with long procedural time and high rates of radiation exposure to patients and operators alike. This has resulted in several occupational concerns. The known risks of radiation exposure are an inherent danger. The Brain Radiation Exposure and Attenuation During Invasive Cardiology Procedures (BRAIN) study demonstrated that radiation exposure is significantly higher on the left and center of the cranium than on the right.[11] Furthermore, brain and neck tumors occurring in a cohort of interventional physicians has been reported, with a high burden in the typically exposed left side of the head.[4] There are further data that, when compared with standard controls, experienced interventional operators have a significantly increased risk of lens opacification.[3] The heavy lead aprons worn to protect against the risks of radiation exposure also pose hazards. Nearly 50% of interventional physicians report a job-related orthopedic injury.[5] There is also an increased risk of hypertension, hypercholesterolemia, and vascular disease among interventional physicians.[2] R-PCI is a novel strategy to reduce the full impact of these hazards by addressing the root cause; that is, radiation exposure. By distancing and shielding the operator, both the stochastic and deterministic effects of radiation exposure are significantly reduced, thus eliminating the need to wear leaded garments and reducing the secondary risk of orthopedic injury.

USE OF THE CorPath ROBOTIC PLATFORM
Patient and Procedure Selection

The decision to perform a robotic procedure can be made before a planned intervention or ad hoc at the time of the completion of diagnostic angiography. In either case, nearly any PCI can be approached robotically. The platform is compatible with all length 0.014-in coronary guidewires, including wires of any composition (eg, coiled, braided, jacketed). The robotic platform is not compatible for independent use with devices that are not rapid exchange (RX) or only over-the-wire (OTW). As such, the catheter used must have an RX port. A rigid proximal hypotube that is kink-resistant and crush-resistant is recommended to reduce the risk of damage when introducing equipment. Given the requirement for devices with an RX lumen, cases in which certain interventional techniques are required may be considered for planned partial robotic procedure with traditional manual completion. Examples of these are complex chronic total occlusions requiring the use of OTW microcatheters to facilitate multiple wire exchanges or severely calcified lesions in which an OTW atherectomy device is required for intervention. In these instances, the portions of the procedure that cannot be performed completely robotically may be performed manually or partially robotically at the tableside.

Procedural Setup

The initial robotic platform, the CorPath 200, was approved for clinical use by the US Food and Drug Administration (FDA) in 2012. The 2 main components are a robotic arm mounted on the catheterization table siderail and a radiation-shielded interventional cockpit located within the catheterization laboratory (Fig. 1). The robotic arm contains a drive platform that houses a single-use sterile cassette. The cassette is manually connected to the guide catheter following coronary artery engagement. When connected, the cassette can accept a 0.014-in guidewire and an RX balloon or stent catheter through grooves within the system (Fig. 2). The arm is electronically connected via cable to the interventional cockpit, behind which the operator sits and controls 2 separate joysticks to manipulate the wire and catheter independently. The newest generation, CorPath GRX, obtained FDA approval for human use in 2016. It contains 3 joysticks: 1 to rotate, advance, and retract the guide catheter; 1 to advance and retract the RX catheter; and 1 to rotate, advance, and retract the guidewire. Cockpit monitors display live fluoroscopic images and hemodynamic data (Fig. 3).

In planned robotic interventions, arterial access must be obtained and a side-arm vascular introducer sheath must be introduced in the typical manual fashion. This can be performed by the primary operator or a trained secondary operator. Access can be either radial or femoral. These approaches have been compared with each other and no differences were noted in regard to procedural outcomes.[12] A guide catheter is then used to engage the coronary artery

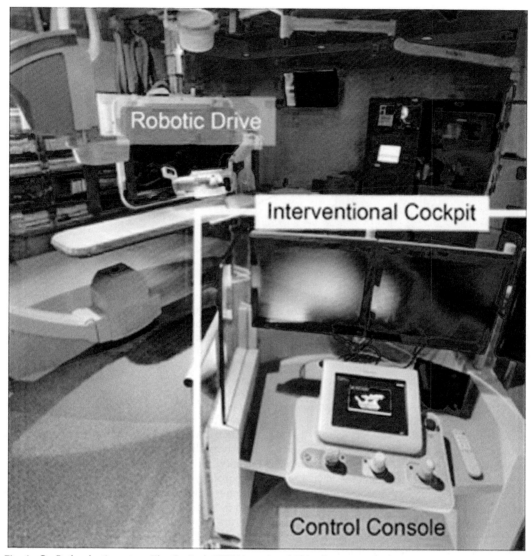

Fig. 1. CorPath robotic system. The CorPath GRX (shown) and 200 robotic systems feature 2 main components: (1) a robotic arm mounted on the catheterization table side rail and (2) a radiation-shielded interventional cockpit with control console. The robotic arm contains a drive platform that houses a single-use sterile cassette. (*Courtesy of Corindus Vascular Robotics, Inc., Waltham, MA.*)

of interest in a typical manual fashion. The guide catheter is then connected to a bleed-back control valve and the combined system is attached to the CorPath GRX system. The guide catheter and bleed-back control valve are placed into the guide catheter gear of the robotic cassette. This allows for rotational control of the unit by the robotic operator. The guide catheter and introducer sheath are connected to a sheath retainer that also allows for advancement and retraction by the robotic operator. A wire is then loaded into the guide catheter, as would be typically done, and an RX catheter is advanced along the wire. After both are safely within the guide catheter, the wire and RX catheter hypotube are independently connected to the cassette, allowing for the advancement and retraction of each individual component by the robotic operator. Of note, improper advancement of the balloon catheter ahead of the wire can occur as a result of failure of precise movement by the operator, as well as secondary to the wire becoming attached to the small magnets within the robotic cassette and failing to advance appropriately. In the authors' experiences, fully advancing the guidewire before advancing the RX balloon catheter over the fixed guidewire has reduced this occurrence.

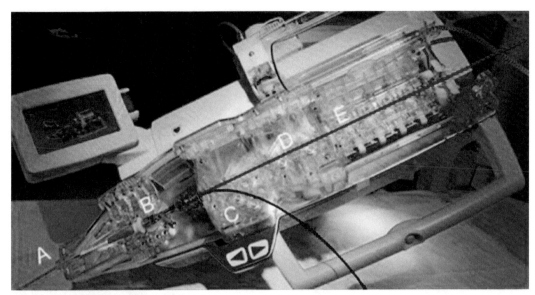

Fig. 2. CorPath GRX drive platform and robotic cassette. During R-PCI using the CorPath GRX system, the guide catheter is encapsulated within the support track (A) and positioned in the Y-connecter holder (B). Here the drive gear allows rotation of the guide catheter. A 0.014-in guidewire is positioned within the center guidewire track (*red line*) and manipulated by drivers facilitating wire advancement or retraction (D) and rotation (E). An RX device is advanced over the guidewire and its proximal support shaft positioned in the linear drive track (*blue line*). Additional drivers facilitate advancement or retraction of the RX catheter (C). (*Courtesy of* Corindus Vascular Robotics, Inc., Waltham, MA.)

Performing Robotic-Assisted Percutaneous Coronary Intervention

Basic approach

A basic R-PCI procedure is performed much along the same lines as a manual procedure. After the guidewire and RX catheter have been loaded into the guide catheter and attached to the robotic cassette, the primary operator may leave the tableside and sit at the CorPath GRX control cockpit. The guidewire is then advanced through the guide catheter and into the coronary artery by pushing up on the guidewire control joystick. If the wire requires retraction, this may be done by pushing down on the joystick. The wire may also be directed during advancement and retraction by rotating the joystick in the corresponding direction. In this manner, the wire is safely navigated through coronary anatomy, across the target lesion, and positioned distally within the vessel. Following wire placement, the previously loaded RX balloon catheter can also be advanced. Standard speed advancement is performed by pushing upward on the catheter joystick and rapid advancement is performed by simultaneously pressing the turbo button on the console. After the balloon is positioned across the target lesion of interest, a tableside assistant is able to manually inflate and deflate the balloon by using extension tubing and lead shielding to reduce his or her own risk of radiation exposure. Balloon removal is performed by pressing downward on the joystick, with rapid removal performed by concurrently pressing the turbo button. Connecting, advancing, positioning, and deploying a coronary stent is performed in the same manner. Flow assessment via pressure wires and RX pressure catheters can also be done using the connecting and advancing methods previously described.

Robotic lesion length determination

The CorPath GRX software contains patented technology that allows for robotic lesion length determination. This is performed by advancing the distal balloon marker to the distal target lesion border. The balloon position counter on the cockpit touchscreen is then zeroed, and the balloon catheter retracted until the distal marker reaches the proximal target lesion border. The balloon counter will report the distance traversed by the balloon as an estimate of lesion length. Notably, this assumes a 1:1 input to movement responsiveness of the system. Measurement can also be performed during advancement of the balloon; however, this has been found to be less reliable due to system responsiveness. Additionally, the same can be performed using the guidewire if a proximal and distal reference point can be identified.

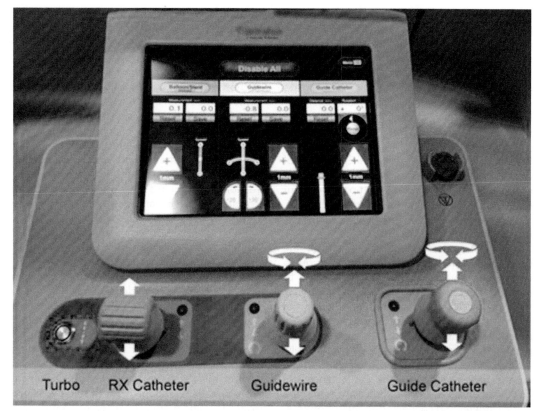

Fig. 3. Robotic cockpit controls for CorPath GRX system. Joysticks controlling the RX catheter (*left*), 0.014-in guidewire (*middle*) and guide catheter (*right*) can all be pushed up to advance and pulled down to retract their respective devices. Guidewire and guide catheter joysticks can be rotated in clockwise or counterclockwise directions to provide device torque control. Depressing the turbo button (*far left*) with simultaneous joystick actuation allows rapid movement of the RX device and guidewire. The guide catheter cannot be rapidly manipulated. (*Courtesy of* Corindus Vascular Robotics, Inc., Waltham, MA.)

Guidewire resistance and robotic advancement

Often, it can be an arduous task to cross lesions, particularly type C, with a guidewire. In these instances, there are robotic maneuvers that can be used to facilitate the crossing of a lesion. The tip of the RX balloon catheter can be advanced robotically toward the guidewire tip to increase tip support and torque response, and to decrease guidewire body friction. This may also assist in robotically redirecting the guidewire before advancing across a lesion. The primary guidewire can also be left in the robotic accessory track while a new guidewire and catheter combination is advanced. Alternatively, the guidewire can be removed and manually exchanged for a specialty guidewire (eg, jacketed, tapered) for use as the primary guidewire in robotic crossing and for subsequent PCI.

A recent development of note is the FDA approval of the CorPath GRX proprietary software called Rotate on Retract. This software allows automatic wire rotation to be performed by the robotic platform during wire retraction. The software uses artificial intelligence in this rotation and is autonomous, acting independently of the operator to facilitate wire passage during subsequent advancement. The primary operator, however, maintains procedural control and is still able to rotate the guidewire as necessary using the cockpit joystick.

Rapid-exchange device resistance

After lesion crossing with the guidewire, there may be resistance to attempts to advance the RX balloon or stent catheter robotically across the lesion. Typically, subtle changes in guidewire position to improve support, or to change the lesion and device interaction, with repeated attempts at crossing are successful. Should this not prove to be the case, a low-profile balloon catheter may be used first for delivery across the lesion and for initial angioplasty to ensure adequate lesion preparation. It is also advisable that highly deliverable contemporary catheters be used during R-PCI. More complicated robotic maneuvers can also be used to facilitate lesion crossing. Quickly pushing the balloon catheter joystick up and pulling down while fixing the guidewire joystick in place mimics the jiggling or knocking that is often done manually. Similarly, simultaneously advancing the balloon catheter while briefly and rapidly retracting the guidewire mimics the rail guidewire position that can be performed manually. One must, of course, be cautious not to retract the guidewire proximal to the balloon catheter tip, or even out of the artery entirely, while using this technique.

Guide catheter manipulation

The newest generation robotic platform, the CorPath GRX, has the added feature of guide catheter manipulation. The operator is able to advance, retract, and rotate the guide catheter through joystick manipulation, with much the same effect as a bedside operator. Notably, advancement and retraction, performed by pushing up or down on the joystick, respectively, moves devices that are connected through the robotic cassette system. Thus, for instance, if a guidewire and a balloon catheter are within the guide catheter and connected to the robotic system, advancement of the guide catheter will advance all 3 devices together. Subtle manipulation of the guide catheter has the effect of moving the guide catheter with minimal change in the location of other devices. The tactile feedback typically noticed during manual PCI is absent when using the robotic platform; therefore, all manipulation must be performed with the utmost caution to prevent excessive movement and potential device dislodgement or even coronary artery damage. With regard to guide catheter rotation, unlike advancement and retraction, there is often a notable delay between operator joystick input and robotic rotation of the guide catheter at the hub. Thus, slow, careful rotation is advised.

In instances during which advancement of a device causes disengagement of the guide catheter from the coronary ostia, reversal of the prior maneuver will typically reengage the equipment. Similarly, removal of a balloon catheter or guidewire may cause deep intubation of the guide catheter. This interplay can be used to safely and successfully maneuver equipment with difficult lesions; for example, a subtle advancement of the balloon catheter before removal to slightly dislodge the guide catheter, followed by retraction of the balloon catheter with subsequent reengagement.

Should it become necessary to advance the guide catheter relative to the coronary artery truly independent of other devices within the system, this can be performed. A brief simultaneous manipulation of the guide catheter in 1 direction and guidewire or balloon catheter in the opposite direction effectively creates a fixed system. To fully fix the devices in place with regard to the coronary artery, the guide catheter joystick must be manipulated in 1 direction and the balloon catheter and guidewire joysticks simultaneously manipulated in the opposite direction. This requires all 3 joysticks be activated concurrently, an advanced level task that is rarely necessary.

CLINICAL EXPERIENCE

The robotic platform has been studied in several prospective series and clinical trials. The first of these, published in 2011, was a first-in-human study demonstrating the safety of the CorPath 200 for use in coronary interventions.[13] This led to the development of the evaluation of the safety and effectiveness of the CorPath 200 System in the Percutaneous Robotically-Enhanced Coronary Intervention (PRECISE) study, a prospective, single-arm, multicenter, safety and feasibility study of R-PCI.[8] In this study, 164 subjects underwent R-PCI on mostly simple coronary lesions (87.2% type A). Clinical success was defined as completion of the planned intervention with less than 30% residual stenosis and the absence of a major adverse cardiac event (MACE). Technical success was defined as successful intracoronary retraction and advancement of the PCI devices by the robotic system without conversion to a manual approach. In the PRECISE study, the clinical success rate was 97.6% and the technical success rate was 98.8%, demonstrating that, in mainly simple lesions, R-PCI was a safe and effective means of intervention.

Subsequently, the Complex Robotically Assisted Percutaneous Coronary Intervention (CORA-PCI) trial was conducted and published in 2017.[9] This single-center trial enrolled all consecutive subjects undergoing PCI, either with the robotic platform (CorPath 200) or in the typical manual fashion, over an 18-month period, during which 103 subjects underwent 108 R-PCI procedures compared with 210 subjects undergoing 226 manual interventions. Using the previous definition, immediate clinical success was 99.1% with both R-PCI and manual PCI. Technical success was defined as completion of the procedure robotically or with partial manual assistance,

Table 1
CorPath 200 or GRX system and compatibility with common interventional devices

Compatible Devices	Partially Compatible Devices	Noncompatible Devices
Coronary guidewire 0.014-in diameter of varying lengths and composition	Nonrotational intravascular ultrasound catheter with RX port, such as Eagle Eye (Volcano, San Diego, CA, USA)	Any OTW catheter, such as a chronic total occlusion microcatheter, or rotational or orbital atherectomy catheter
RX balloon or stent catheter with rigid proximal hypotube	• Susceptible to crushing or kinking, poor robotic control, and image degradation	Any rotation-based intravascular imaging catheter, such as Opticross
• A secondary wire and catheter can be robotically manipulated while primary devices are maintained (and manually manipulated) in a passive accessory track	Laser atherectomy catheter with RX port, such as ELCA (Philips, Andover, MA)	IVUS (Boston Scientific, Marlborough, MA), Revolution or Refinity (Volcano), or Dragonfly
• A jailed side-branch wire can be maintained in the accessory track but resistance to removal may overwhelm the robotic drive	• Susceptible to crushing or kinking, poor robotic control, and ineffective laser transmission	(Abbott Vascular, Santa Clara, CA)
• A secondary balloon or stent catheter can be maintained and manually manipulated in the accessory track for intervention of bifurcation lesions	Guide catheter extenders	Distal embolic protection device deployment and retrieval catheter
	• Manually inserted and manipulated but can be maintained in the accessory track	
	Distal embolic filter wires	
	• Manually deployed and retrieved	
	• Robotically held in place during intervention	

and freedom from a MACE. This was achieved in 91.5% of the R-PCI cohort, which comprised mostly complex lesions (78.3% type B2/C lesions). Furthermore, 92.6% of cases were completed either entirely robotically or with partial manual assistance. At 12 months, long-term clinical outcomes between the R-PCI and the manual cohorts were found to be the same.[10]

The Post-Market CorPath Registry on the CorPath 200 System in Percutaneous Coronary Interventions (PRECISION) study, the results of which were presented in 2017, compared radial versus femoral access in subjects undergoing R-PCI using the CorPath 200 system.[14] Performed with multiple operators at 16 centers across the United States, the study comprised 452 procedures performed from a transradial approach and 298 from a transfemoral approach; 949 lesions were intervened on, 63.4% were type B2/C. Technical success, defined as procedural success with less than 30% residual stenosis without manual assistance and without an in-hospital MACE, was achieved in 88.6% of the radial procedures and 82.4% of the femoral procedures. Clinical success, defined as procedural success without an in-hospital MACE, was achieved in 98.9% of the radial cases and 94.9% of the femoral cases. Propensity-adjusted analysis identified

no difference between either approach, indicating both to be safe, feasible, and effective.

A recent study was the first to use the new-generation CorPath GRX system. This demonstrated first-in-human safety and efficacy of the new platform in complex coronary lesions (77.3% type B2/C).[15] The clinical success rate of 97.5% was similar to the first-generation system.[13] Of these cases, 90.0% were completed entirely robotically, an improvement from the first-generation system, reflecting the expanded capabilities of the CorPath GRX system.

The reasons for technical failure when using the R-PCI have been elucidated in these studies. A planned, manual-assistance approach has been used for interventions, such as those requiring an embolic protection device, or for intravascular imaging, such as intravascular ultrasound. These devices, although theoretically compatible with a complete robotic approach, are cumbersome and difficult to use entirely robotically and, as such, a hybrid procedure is often preferred (Table 1). The CorPath 200 was limited in its ability to manipulate the guide catheter, which was ultimately the reason for manual assistance in 40% of the cases requiring a partial manual approach.[16] The CorPath GRX directly addresses this issue. In the CorPath GRX feasibility study, all technical failures were directly

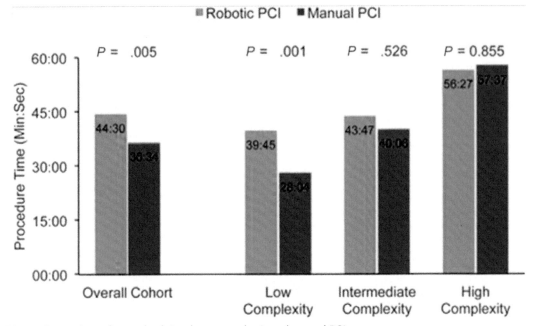

Fig. 4. Comparison of procedural time between robotic and manual PCI.

related to complex anatomic disease with no guide catheter disengagement in the cohort.[15] Adverse events and overall inadequate support are thus the primary issues one faces when attempting a robotic approach that may require partial or complete manual conversion.

The demonstrated safety and efficacy of R-PCI within the coronary vasculature has opened the door for various other aspects of cardiovascular interventions. The Robotic-Assisted Peripheral Intervention for Peripheral Arterial Disease (RAPID) study was a prospective, single-arm, single-center, open-label, nonrandomized study of robotic-assisted peripheral vascular interventions. A total of 20 subjects with symptomatic peripheral arterial disease (Rutherford class 2–5) affecting the femoropopliteal artery were enrolled. Device technical success, safety, and clinical procedural success were achieved in all subjects, demonstrating the feasibility and safety of using a robotic-assisted platform for performing peripheral arterial revascularization and leading to FDA approval of the device for peripheral interventions.[17] Compatibility with other wire sizes, including 0.018-in and 0.035-in diameters, could expand the utility of the robotic system in peripheral interventions. Ergonomic and radiation safety challenges experienced by peripheral vascular operators may be overcome by the combination of enhanced guidewire and OTW catheter compatibility.

Further data stemming from these studies demonstrate the significant reduction in operator radiation exposure with the robotic system compared with manual PCI. In the PRECISE study, radiation exposure was reduced 95.2% between the shielded interventional cockpit of the CorPath system when compared with simultaneously measured bedside exposure.[8] The CORA-PCI trial found that, even in complex lesions, the overall fluoroscopy time and dose-area-product measurements between R-PCI and manual PCI were not different in a propensity-matched analysis, indicating no increase in exposure to the patient.[9] Overall procedure time in the CORA-PCI trial was found to be higher within the R-PCI patient cohort. Notably, however, this was driven by a statistically significant increase in procedural time for simple lesions in the study. Those lesions of moderate or high complexity had overall procedure times that were equivalent between the R-PCI and the manual PCI cohorts (Fig. 4).[9] Contrast utilization was also the same between the 2 groups.

LIMITATIONS OF ROBOTIC PERCUTANEOUS CORONARY INTERVENTION

As previously noted, R-PCI has been shown to be safe and effective for both simple and complex coronary interventions. Several system limitations do exist. Poor guidewire and guide catheter support were the leading reasons for robotic failure and subsequent manual operator input during interventions on complex lesions within the CORA-PCI study. Other reasons for conversion included the use of interventional devices or techniques beyond the capabilities of the robotic platform and, rarely, adverse events. This study, however, used the older CorPath 200 system. The CorPath GRX helps address the guide catheter support issue by allowing operator manipulation from the robotic cockpit. As an example, ostial right coronary lesions were previously not feasible from a robotic perspective given the need to repeatedly advance and retract the guide catheter during stent deployment; this is now possible with the new CorPath GRX system. Lesions that are difficult to cross and suboptimal support from intracoronary devices do, however, remain an issue. As such, in cases that seem to have complex anatomy or other concerning features, it is imperative to choose appropriately sized and supportive guides and devices for intervention. Guide catheter extensions can also be manually positioned before robotic intervention for additional support.

Other interventional scenarios require partial or complete manual operation during intervention. This includes planned bifurcation stenting because the CorPath system is not currently able to simultaneously control and manipulate multiple wires and catheters. A provisional approach is possible; however, partial assistance is required for manipulation of the second balloon during any planned, concurrent balloon inflations. This hybrid approach uses the robot to position 1 guidewire and balloon or stent catheter at a time while final simultaneous balloon or stent positioning is achieved with combined robotic and manual input with assistance from a second tableside operator. Vein graft intervention using a distal embolic protection device also requires manual input to deploy and retrieve the filter. The remainder of the procedure, including the primary wiring of the vessel before filter placement, can be done from a robotic approach because the system is capable of holding the distal device in place during balloon or stent manipulation. Revascularization of chronic total occlusions can be completed robotically. This is limited, however, in the inability to use OTW systems, and is best suited for less complex occlusions thought to be achievable by an antegrade wire escalation approach.

Debulking of severely calcified lesions or lesions containing significant in-stent restenosis is capable of being performed robotically, although there may be significant limitations. Rotational and orbital atherectomy devices are incompatible with the robotic system. RX laser atherectomy catheters, such as ELCA (Spectranetics, Colorado Springs, CO, USA), are partially compatible with the robotic systems but are susceptible to damage during use. Intravascular imaging is possible using the robotic system but, as with atherectomy, may be limited. Multiphased array intravascular ultrasound, such as Eagle Eye Platinum (Volcano Corporation, San Diego, CA, USA), does not use rotating components. As with laser atherectomy catheters, this is susceptible to damage during R-PCI but remains a feasible alternative. Rotating intravascular imaging devices, such as single-array intravascular ultrasound and optical coherence tomography catheters, are also incompatible with the CorPath platform owing to the potential for catheter damage.

DISCUSSION AND FUTURE DIRECTIONS

There are emerging data for R-PCI in the complex, high-risk (and indicated) population (CHIP). A total of 6 subjects from the PRECISION registry underwent left main R-PCI, with or without hemodynamic support, with complete procedural success.[18] CHIP interventions often have prolonged procedural times, resulting in higher radiation exposure of the patient and physician, with the added potential for operator fatigue. R-PCI could potentially mitigate these issues. As previously noted, laser atherectomy is an adjunctive lesion modification modality that can be implemented in the second-generation robotic system using the RX feature of the ELCA catheter. This implementation, specific to the robotic system, provides precise control of the atherectomy catheter, ensuring that the laser catheter is advanced in a controlled manner (rate of 0.5–1.0 mm) that is maintained for the duration of atherectomy.[19] The use of R-PCI for the management of ST-elevation myocardial infarction has been described as a case report; however, larger studies are lacking.[20]

The contemporary robotic platform is still an emerging technology and has certain design limitations. These include but are not limited to the single set of drives that are used. A second set of drives controlling dual guidewires and catheters would allow completely robotic intervention of bifurcation lesions. It may also address suboptimal guide catheter support with easy introduction and positioning of a second wire. The incompatibility of OTW devices, and the physical tethering of the robotic arm to the interventional table and controls are also shortcomings of the current system. Furthermore, the resource utilization associated with R-PCI compared with traditional PCI remains unknown.

The possible untethering of the robotic arm from interventional controls through high-speed secure wireless data transfer could be the most impactful advancement for R-PCI. This would allow a single operator to control remote robotic arms (eg, in different laboratories, buildings, or cities) with local assistance. The feasibility of remote R-PCI, or telestenting, was recently demonstrated in a small prospective subject cohort[21] in which the robotic cockpit was located in an isolated room outside the catheterization laboratory and the procedure conducted via audio-visual communication with the laboratory staff. Nineteen out of 20 procedures were successfully completed, with no deaths or urgent revascularization occurring before discharge; the procedure has now been done from 100 miles away in a pig model.[22] Relocation of the interventional controls out of the laboratory entirely could allow elimination of a shielded cockpit altogether. Larger studies confirming telestenting safety and feasibility across greater geographic distances and overcoming basic technological hurdles will be needed before attempting R-PCI across state lines or national borders.

SUMMARY

The recent application and advancement of robotic systems have made an impressive impact on interventional cardiology in regard to procedural efficiency, operator radiation reduction, and safety. With future improvements overcoming the need for manual assistance and incompatibility with some devices, and the expansion of robotic applicability for coronary and noncoronary interventions, this technology will play a major role in the future of interventional cardiology.

REFERENCES

1. Gruntzig AR, Senning A, Siegenthaler WE. Nonoperative dilatation of coronary-artery stenosis: percutaneous transluminal coronary angioplasty. N Engl J Med 1979;301:61–8.
2. Andreassi MG, Piccaluga E, Guagliumi G, et al. Occupational health risks in cardiac catheterization laboratory workers. Circ Cardiovasc Interv 2016;9: e003273.
3. Karatasakis A, Brilakis HS, Danek BA, et al. Radiation-associated lens changes in the cardiac catheterization laboratory: results from the IC-CATARACT (CATaracts Atttributed to Radiation in the CaTh lab) study. Catheter Cardiovasc Interv 2018;91(4):647–54.
4. Roguin A, Goldstein J, Bar O, et al. Brain and neck tumors among physicians performing interventional procedures. Am J Cardiol 2013;111:1368–72.
5. Klein LW, Tra Y, Garratt KN, et al, Society for Cardiovascular Angiography and Interventions. Occupational health hazards of interventional cardiologists in the current decade: results of the 2014 SCAI membership survey. Catheter Cardiovasc Interv 2015;86:913–24.
6. Kwoh YS, Hou J, Jonckheere EA, et al. A robot with improved absolute positioning accuracy for CT guided stereotactic brain surgery. IEEE Trans Biomed Eng 1988;35:153–61.
7. Pourdjabbar A, Ang L, Behnamfar O, et al. Robotics in percutaneous cardiovascular interventions. Expert Rev Cardiovasc Ther 2017;15:825–33.
8. Weisz G, Metzger DC, Caputo RP, et al. Safety and feasibility of robotic percutaneous coronary intervention: PRECISE (Percutaneous Robotically-Enhanced Coronary Intervention) study. J Am Coll Cardiol 2013;61:1596–600.
9. Mahmud E, Naghi J, Ang L, et al. Demonstration of the Safety and Feasibility of Robotically Assisted Percutaneous Coronary Intervention in Complex Coronary Lesions: Results of the CORA-PCI study (Complex Robotically Assisted Percutaneous Coronary Intervention). JACC Cardiovasc Interv 2017; 10(13):1320–7.
10. Walters DC, Reeves RR, Patel MP, et al. Complex robotic compared to manual coronary interventions: 6- and 12-month outcomes. Catheter Cardiovasc Interv 2018. [Epub ahead of print].
11. Reeves RR, Ang L, Bahadorani J, et al. Invasive Cardiologists Are Exposed to Greater Left Sided Cranial Radiation: The BRAIN Study (Brain Radiation Exposure and Attenuation During Invasive Cardiology Procedures). JACC Cardiovasc Interv 2015;8(9):1197–206.
12. Smitson C, Ang L, Reeves R, et al. Safety and feasibility of a novel, second generation robotic-assisted system for percutaneous coronary intervention: first-in-human report. J Am Coll Cardiol 2017;70:B55–6.
13. Granada JF, Delgado JA, Uribe MP, et al. First-in-human evaluation of a novel robotic-assisted coronary angioplasty system. JACC Cardiovasc Interv 2011;4:460–5.
14. Mahmud E. Efficacy and safety outcomes of radial-versus femoral-access robotic percutaneous coronary intervention: final results of the multicenter PRECISION registry. Society for Cardiovascular Angiography and Interventions 2017 Scientific

Sessions. 2017. Available at: http://www.scai.org/Press/detail.aspx?cid=eb588694-bc51-4552-b8c9-6b50c6daff87#.W6Qnqv6WyUl. Accessed May 11, 2017.

15. Smitson C, Ang L, Reeves R, et al. Safety and feasibility of a novel, second generation robotic-assisted system for percutaneous coronary intervention: first-in-human report. J Invasive Cardiol 2018;30(4):152–6.

16. Harrison J, Ang L, Naghi J, et al. Robotically-assisted percutaneous coronary intervention: reasons for partial manual assistance or manual conversion. Cardiovasc Revasc Med 2018;19(5 Pt A):526–31.

17. Mahmud E, Schmid F, Kalmar P, et al. Feasibility and safety of robotic peripheral vascular interventions: results of the rapid trial. JACC Cardiovasc Interv 2016;9(19):2058–64.

18. Mahmud E, Dominguez A, Bahadorani J. First-in-human robotic percutaneous coronary intervention for unprotected left main stenosis. Catheter Cardiovasc Interv 2016;88(4):565–70.

19. Almasoud A, Walters D, Mahmud E. Robotically performed excimer laser coronary atherectomy: proof of feasibility. Catheter Cardiovasc Interv 2018;92(4):713–6.

20. Kapur V, Smilowitz NR, Weisz G. Complex robotic-enhanced coronary intervention. Catheter Cardiovasc Interv 2018;83:915–21.

21. Madder RD, VanOosterhout SM, Jacoby ME, et al. Percutaneous coronary intervention using a combination of robotics and telecommunications by an operator in a separate physical location from the patient: an early exploration into the feasibility of telestenting (the remote-pci study). EuroIntervention 2017;12(13):1569–76.

22. Aller D. Operator performs robot assisted PCI from 100 miles away. Cardiovascular Business. 2018. Available at: https://www.cardiovascularbusiness.com/topics/coronary-intervention-surgery/operator-performs-pci-100-miles-away. Accessed July 19, 2018.

Orbital Atherectomy
A Comprehensive Review

Evan Shlofmitz, DO[a], Richard Shlofmitz, MD[b], Michael S. Lee, MD[c],*

KEYWORDS

- Orbital atherectomy • Percutaneous coronary intervention • Atherectomy
- Calcified coronary lesion • Coronary artery calcification

KEY POINTS

- Severely calcified lesions can inhibit adequate stent expansion.
- Inadequate stent expansion is associated with poor clinical outcomes.
- Orbital atherectomy facilitates lesion preparation to maximize stent expansion.

INTRODUCTION

Coronary artery calcification (CAC) negatively affects clinical outcomes after percutaneous coronary intervention (PCI).[1,2] Despite significant advances in device technology and techniques within interventional cardiology, CAC remains a central challenge to achieving optimal results with revascularization. Heavily calcified lesions are increasingly encountered during PCI.

Coronary Artery Calcification

Advanced age, diabetes, chronic kidney disease, and tobacco use all are associated with increased prevalence of CAC. The degree of CAC is associated with the impact on PCI. CAC can impede successful stent delivery and is associated with increased adverse events both short and long term. Acutely during PCI, CAC is associated with increased vessel dissection, vessel perforation, malapposed stent struts, and underexpanded stents.[3] Long term, CAC is linked to increased risk of stent thrombosis, restenosis, and major adverse cardiac events (MACE).[4,5] Increased target lesion revascularization (TLR) is influenced from a combination of reduced drug concentration and uptake into the vessel from drug-eluting stents combined with stent underexpansion.[6] One of the most important predictors of outcomes after drug-eluting stent implantation is final minimal stent area.[7–9] The larger the final stent area is, the better the outcomes. To maximize stent size in a heavily calcified lesion, typically requires modifying the plaque morphology before stent implantation.

CAC is significantly underappreciated and underdiagnosed on routine coronary angiography. Mintz and colleagues[10] demonstrated that while angiography revealed calcium in 38% of lesions, intravascular ultrasound (IVUS) detected calcium in 73% of lesions. These findings from more than 2 decades ago were corroborated recently in an IVUS and optical coherence tomography (OCT) study, which found significant underdetection of calcium by angiography compared with IVUS or OCT.[11] If CAC is unrecognized, appropriate treatment cannot be applied. For this reason, the authors advocate liberal use of intravascular imaging to comprehensively assess lesions and guide the intervention as needed.

Treatment Options

Severe CAC acutely poses 2 main issues during PCI: the ability to deliver a stent and the ability

---

Disclosure Statement: R. Shlofmitz has a consulting agreement with Cardiovascular Systems, Inc.
[a] MedStar Washington Hospital Center, 110 Irving Street, Suite 4B1, Washington, DC 20010, USA; [b] St. Francis Hospital- The Heart Center, 100 Port Washington Boulevard, Suite 105, Roslyn, NY 11576, USA; [c] UCLA Medical Center, 100 Medical Plaza Suite 630, Los Angeles, CA 90095, USA
* Corresponding author.
E-mail address: mslee@mednet.ucla.edu

2211-7458/19/© 2018 Elsevier Inc. All rights reserved.

to achieve complete stent expansion. These limitations have been addressed by several devices and treatment strategies. Treatment options include atherectomy (rotational, orbital, or laser) or specialty balloons (cutting, scoring, or high pressure), with alternative modalities incorporating percutaneous lithoplasty under clinical investigation. Utilization of atherectomy devices with PCI varies widely and has been reported to range from 3% to 18%.[12,13] Data on the rates of utilization of orbital atherectomy specifically however are limited.

Guidelines

Orbital atherectomy (OA) is the first device specifically approved for routine lesion preparation before stent implantation. The 2011 American College of Cardiology/American Heart Association PCI guidelines provide a class IIa, level of evidence C recommendation for rotational atherectomy (RA) in heavily calcified lesions that may be difficult to cross or dilate. However, the guidelines recommend against routine use of RA (class III, level of evidence A).[14] Society guidelines for revascularization have not been updated since approval of OA, and as such the guidelines do not make specific recommendations regarding the use of OA. Nonetheless, it is a major change in revascularization strategy to go from a bail-out atherectomy approach, to an up-front treatment technique. The focus has shifted from the use of atherectomy for simply to facilitate stent delivery in difficult to cross lesions, to lesion preparation to optimize stent results and maximize final stent expansion. The goal with lesion preparation is not to cross the lesion; rather, it is to modify the plaque and change its morphology and compliance to maximize the likelihood of achieving adequate stent expansion. Understanding this paradigm shift in treatment evolution from debulking of plaque to lesion modification is vital. OA can be used accordingly to tailor therapy to obtain the best possible results.[15]

Device Description

The Diamondback 360 Coronary orbital atherectomy system (OAS) (Cardiovascular Systems, Inc., Saint Paul, MN, USA) consists of a drive shaft with a diamond-coated crown that is eccentrically mounted and ablates calcified plaque as it comes into contact with a lesion.[16] Differential sanding permits healthy tissue to flex away from the crown during orbit. There is a tableside, electric-powered motor handle, with speed selection options for low speed (80,000 rpm), high speed (120,000 rpm), or

GlideAssist (5000 rpm) (Fig. 1). The classic crown consists of a 1.25 mm burr that can sand bidirectionally over a 0.012″ (0.014″ tip) ViperWire coronary guidewire. Device setup is quick, and the system can be safely controlled by a single operator.[17]

Owing to the eccentric mounting, the crown's orbit expands elliptically via centrifugal force and can achieve a maximum lumen diameter greater than 1.8 mm.[18] The bidirectional mechanism can reduce the likelihood of burr entrapment. The average particle size created by OA is 2.04 μm, which is smaller than a red blood cell.[19] ViperSlide lubricant (Cardiovascular Systems, Inc., Saint Paul, MN, USA) must be infused during device use, and a bag containing 20 mL ViperSlide per liter of saline can be attached to an intravenous pole-mounted OAS pump that delivers the lubricant. The elliptical orbit permits continuous flow of saline and blood during treatment. Continuous flow, combined with small particle size, has been theorized to contribute to the low rates of thermal injury, transient heart block, and no reflow seen with OA.[20,21] A 6-french or larger guide is required for use. OA treatment techniques and best practices have previously been described in detail.[18]

Treatment with OA is a time-dependent therapy. The slower the burr is advanced through the lesion, the larger the luminal gain can be achieved, with an ideal speed of 1 to 3 mm/s. A 1:1 movement with the crown and advancer knob must always be maintained. Consistent and slow advancement of the burr is essential to optimize results. Treatment of calcified lesions with OA leads to ablation of calcified tissue with luminal gain.[22] The modest luminal gain from debulking, however, is not the main goal of treatment. Plaque modification together with calcium fractures from lesion preparation with OA can facilitate stent expansion with adjunctive balloon dilatation.[23]

The micro crown is an alternative crown option, which has a diamond-coated tip that allows engagement in ostial or nearly occlusive lesions. The micro crown was evaluated in the prospective, multicenter Coronary Orbital Atherectomy System Study (COAST) trial (NCT02132611), which enrolled 100 patients in the United States and Japan. Initial results from this study indicate procedural success was achieved in 85% of patients, with 22.2% MACE at 1-year follow-up.[24]

When to Consider Orbital Atherectomy

The thickness of calcium highly influences the likelihood of calcium fracture to occur with balloon angioplasty.[25,26] Calcium fracture during

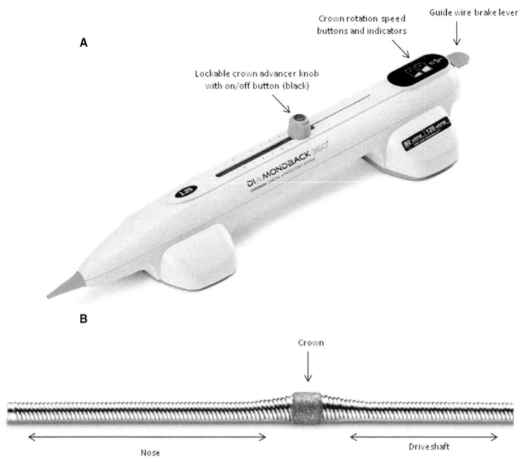

Fig. 1. Diamondback 360 Coronary orbital atherectomy system. (A) Coronary classic orbital atherectomy device. (B) 1.25 mm Classic Crown. (©2018 Cardiovascular Systems, Inc. CSI®, Diamondback 360®, GlideAssist®, ViperWire Advance® and ViperSlide® are registered trademarks of Cardiovascular Systems, Inc., and used with permission.)

PCI of calcified lesions can improve stent expansion. OCT-based data suggest that calcium thickness less than 0.24 mm can predict calcium fracture in lesions treated with only balloon angioplasty before stent implantation.[27] As such, lesions with minimum calcium thickness exceeding this threshold can benefit from atherectomy-induced calcium modification to avoid stent underexpansion.

The ability to fully dilate a calcified lesion is not simply based on calcium thickness. The total calcium burden also plays an important role, and as such factors including length and arc of calcium are also contributors to whether adequate stent expansion can be achieved with angioplasty alone.[3] An OCT-based calcium scoring system has been developed to predict stent expansion, with 2 points for maximum angle greater than 180°, 1 point for maximum thickness greater than 0.5 mm, and 1 point for length greater than 5 mm. On multivariate analysis the calcium score was an independent predictor of stent underexpansion, and lesions with a score less than 3 had excellent stent expansion, and lesions with a score of 4 had poor stent expansion (96% vs 78%, $P<.01$)[28] (Box 1). It is therefore recommended to consider an atherectomy approach whenever a lesions calcium score is 4, to avoid underexpansion.

Treatment Speeds

GlideAssist is a recently added device feature that can be used to assist in advancing and retracting the crown over the guidewire. This speed setting should not be used for lesion treatment.

All treatments with OA should begin with a pass on low speed. Low speed is often adequate for complete lesion preparation. High-speed treatment is not necessary for all lesions. Specifically, high speed should be avoided in highly tortuous vessels or vessels less than 3.0 mm in

> **Box 1**
> **OCT-derived calcium score for prediction of stent underexpansion[28]**
>
> - Maximum calcium angle greater than 180° (2 points)
> - Maximum calcium thickness greater than 0.5 mm (1 point)
> - Calcium length greater than 5 mm (1 point)
>
> Lesions with a calcium score of 4 are at risk for stent underexpansion.

diameter. Escalation to high speed should only occur when inadequate ablation has occurred after 2 treatment passes on low speed. During treatment, a minimum distance exceeding 10 mm should always be maintained between the OA crown and guidewire tip.

Treatment Endpoint

The maximum treatment time per pass should not exceed 30 seconds. An audible alert can be heard after 25 seconds of continuous treatment, indicating that the crown should be moved to a position outside of the lesion. In between treatment passes, a rest period equal to the treatment time should be met at a minimum. For example, if the initial pass lasted 20 seconds, a rest period of 20 seconds should precede the next pass. Longer rest periods may be needed when treating longer lesions, or if there is any evidence of a bradycardic response or hemodynamic changes, to allow time for adequate recovery.

During ablation, tactile and audible changes will be appreciated. When the OA crown is engaging calcified plaque, there is a change in appreciated audible pitch with variable, alternating sound during ablation. Pitch change is reduced as a treatment endpoint has been reached. The treatment endpoint has been reached when pitch change is no longer heard, coupled with a reduction in tactile resistance. A predefined number of treatment passes should not be used. With experience, the tactile and audible feedback will be easily recognized. After treatment with OA, the lesion can be assessed with intravascular imaging to confirm the presence of the characteristic smooth, concave sanding and/or calcium fracture. Alternatively, at the operator's discretion a balloon can be expanded at the lesion to ensure it fully dilates before stent implantation.

Clinical Data

The first-in-human trial assessing OA in coronary arteries was the ORBIT I study, which assessed the safety and feasibility of orbital atherectomy for the treatment of de novo calcified coronary lesions. The prospective, nonrandomized study evaluated the safety and feasibility in 50 patients from 2 sites in India[29] with a mean lesion length of 13.4 mm. Device success was 98%, and procedure success was 94%. Clinical outcomes are summarized in Table 1.

The ORBIT II trial was the US-based investigational device trial that led to Food and Drug Administration (FDA) approval in 2013. ORBIT II was a multicenter, prospective, open-label, single-arm trial enrolling 443 patients from 49 sites with severely calcified de novo coronary disease. Since no other device had specific FDA approval for routine lesion preparation, the study lacked a control arm. The primary endpoint was 30-day MACE using a performance criterion of freedom from 30-day MACE greater than 83%. The investigators found that OA facilitated stent delivery and when compared with historical controls improved clinical outcomes.[35] The device met the prespecified performance criterion (freedom from 30-day MACE, 89.6% [95% confidence interval (CI), 86.7% to 92.5%]). Other

Table 1
Summary of clinical studies

	ORBIT I[29,30]	ORBIT II[31,32]	Real-World Multicenter[33,34]
Number of patients	50	443	458
Dissection	12	3.4	0.9
No reflow/ slow flow	0	0.9	0.7
Perforation	2	1.8	0.7
In-hospital MACE	4	9.8	–
1-y MACE	–	16.4	12.6[b]
1-y cardiac death	–	3.0	4.0[a]
1-y MI	–	9.7	1.8
1-y TVR	–	5.9	7.5
3-y MACE	18.2	23.5	–
3-y cardiac death	9.1	6.7	–
3-y MI	6.1	11.2	–
3-y TVR	–	10.2	–
3-y TLR	3	7.8	

Abbreviations: MI, myocardial infarction; TVR, target vessel revascularization.
[a] Represents rate of all-cause mortality.
[b] Includes cerebrovascular events (1.3%).

procedural and clinical outcomes are summarized in Table 1. At 3-year follow-up, the MACE rate was 23.5%, with cardiac death occurring in 6.7%, myocardial infarction in 11.2%, target vessel revascularization (TVR) in 10.2%, and 7.8% TLR.[31] To put these results of difficult-to-treat patients in perspective, in the ROTATAXUS study of patients with moderate-severe calcification that were treated with RA, MACE at 2-year follow-up occurred in nearly one-third of patients.[36]

The ORBIT series of trials excluded patients with unprotected left main disease and impaired left ventricular systolic function with ejection fraction less than or equal to 25% and chronic kidney disease unless on dialysis. These patients make up a large number of patients with calcified coronary disease that are encountered in real-world practice. As such, the authors investigated the outcome of OA in an all-comer, observational registry comprising 458 patients treated at 3 centers.[33] This registry allowed for the evaluation of OA in patient populations that were not well represented in the ORBIT trials. At 1-year follow-up, major adverse cardiac and cerebrovascular events occurred in 12.6%, mortality in 4.0%, and TVR in 7.5% of patients.[34] Therefore, OA was found to be safe and effective in this complex patient population. The current state of clinical data for OA is summarized in Table 1.

Comparison with Rotational Atherectomy

Several studies have sought to compare outcomes of OA with RA. These studies have largely been retrospective or observational and are summarized in Table 2. Two separate OCT-based studies have compared the 2 modalities to assess their relative mechanisms of action. Yamamoto and colleagues[37] found that in lesions with larger luminal area, OA led to greater plaque modification compared with RA, whereas in lesions with smaller lumen area, a similar degree of plaque modification occurred. Final stent expansion was similar after plaque modification with either device. The OA 1.25 mm burr is capable of effectively treating lumens larger than 1.25 mm in diameter due to the unique orbital mechanism of action. Kini and colleagues[38] also found several important mechanistic differences between the devices. They demonstrated no difference in the incidence of dissections; however, OA resulted in deeper tissue modification and better final stent apposition. A small, randomized trial comparing the 2 modalities is ongoing: the Comparison of Orbital Versus Rotational Atherectomy Effects

On Coronary Microcirculation in PCI [ORACLE] (NCT03021577) will assess the effects of the 2 atherectomy systems on the coronary microcirculation.

Special Populations and Lesions

Studies have assessed the outcomes of OA in several specific patient populations. In the ORBIT II trial, female patients had a higher rate of dissection.[44] Despite this, there was no significant difference in adverse events seen at 30 days compared with male patients. The safety of OA in female patients is supported by real world data, which found no significant sex-based differences in angiographic complications or 30-day outcomes.[45] OA has been demonstrated to be safe in patients with advanced age, a history of diabetes, or prior coronary artery bypass grafts (CABG).[46–48] OA has also shown favorable results in specific lesion subtypes including small vessels (≤2.5 mm), long lesions (≥50 mm), aorto-ostial lesions, and unprotected left main disease.[49–52] Table 3 summarizes the clinical data of OA in specific patient populations.

The Role of Intravascular Imaging

Intravascular imaging has a prominent role in diagnosing and treating calcified lesions. Intravascular imaging is essential to accurately assess the presence, features, and severity of coronary artery calcification and to determine when treatment with OA is warranted. Baseline intravascular imaging assessment detects the extent of calcium, as well as guides appropriate selection of stent size and length. The authors recommend an OCT-guided approach to lesion preparation with orbital atherectomy (Fig. 2). In ORBIT-II, there were significantly fewer stents placed, with increased post-OA minimum lumen diameter in patients with IVUS assessment of the degree of lesion calcification before OA as compared with patients with angiographic assessment of the degree of lesion calcification.[64] With OA specifically, intravascular imaging can confirm adequate plaque modification and assess for the presence of calcium fracture before implanting a stent (Fig. 3). After stent implantation in a calcified lesion, intravascular imaging is vital to ensure adequate stent expansion. Incorporating an algorithmic intravascular imaging–based approach into routine practice can help ensure maximal stent expansion has been safely achieved to help minimize the likeliness of restenosis and stent thrombosis.[65]

Table 2
Studies comparing orbital atherectomy with rotational atherectomy

Clinical Study	Population Studied (N =)	Summary
Yamamoto et al,[37] 2017	OA = 30, RA = 30	OA creates more calcium modification in lesions with larger lumen area as well as more noncalcified plaque modification; the effect in lesions with smaller lumen area is similar between devices. Final stent expansion was similar after plaque modification with either device
Kini et al,[38] 2015	OA = 10, RA = 10	OA resulted in deeper tissue modifications (lacunae) as shown by OCT imaging
Lee et al,[39] 2017	OA = 50, RA = 67	Similar clinical outcomes at 30-d follow-up
Okamoto et al,[40] 2018	OA = 184, RA = 965	OA use was associated with lower unadjusted but similar adjusted 1-y MACE outcomes compared with RA
COAP-PCI,[41] 2018	OA = 273, RA = 273	OA was associated with significantly decreased in-hospital myocardial infarction and mortality after propensity score matching with decreased fluoroscopy time
Koifman et al,[42] 2018	OA = 57, RA = 191	Higher rate of coronary dissections with OA compared with RA, but no difference in periprocedural events
Megaly et al,[43] 2018	OA = 4, RA = 4	No patients experienced bradyarrhythmias with upfront aminophylline administration before atherectomy

Abbreviation: OCT, optical coherence tomography.

Complications

Although uncommon, complications can occur with any device or procedure, and preparation is most important to minimize the impact of a procedural complication and prevent its occurrence. Coronary perforation is among the most serious complication that can occur with OA. The reported incidence with initial experience ranges from 0.7% to 2%.[29,31,33] The management of coronary perforations largely depends on the severity of perforation and its location within the coronary tree. Wire perforations can often be managed with coil embolization, whereas ablation-related perforations typically require a covered stent. Surveillance with echocardiography is important in these patients, with a low threshold for pericardiocentesis in these scenarios. With increased experience, appropriate escalation to high speed, and avoidance of OA within highly tortuous vessels, the occurrence of coronary perforations may be reduced. OA should be avoided in anatomy with greater than 2 bends exceeding 90° angulations, or when evidence of wire wrinkling from tension buildup is present leading to vessel straightening. High speed should be avoided when the vessel diameter is less than 3 mm. Burr advancement should always occur consistently and slowly with a target travel speed of 1 to 3 mm per second.

Table 3
Studies assessing orbital atherectomy in specific populations

Population	ORBIT-II Trial Summary	Real-World Study Summary
Female	Higher rates of dissections in women, with no significant differences in 30-d outcomes[44]	No difference in angiographic complications or 30-d outcomes[45]
Diabetics	Rates of adverse clinical events in diabetic patients who underwent orbital atherectomy were low and similar to nondiabetic patients at 1-y follow-up[47]	Low event rates that were similar to nondiabetics[53,54]
History of CABG	Higher incidence of non-Q-wave MI in patients with CABG at 1 y[48]	Similar angiographic and clinical outcomes at 30 d compared with patients who had no previous history of CABG[55]
Elderly (age ≥75)	Rates of adverse clinical events in elderly patients who underwent orbital atherectomy were low and similar to the nonelderly patients at 30-d and 3-y follow-up[46]	Similar rates of angiographic complications and 30-d adverse events compared with nonelderly patients treated with OA[56]
Impaired ejection fraction	1-y cardiac death was higher in patients with left ventricular systolic dysfunction, however no significant differences in clinical events at 30 d[57]	Plaque modification with OA was safe and well tolerated in patients with systolic dysfunction with higher rates of 30-d clinical adverse events[58]
Chronic kidney disease	Higher MACE rate through 1-y follow-up due to a higher rate of periprocedural MI[59]	No significant differences in MACCE at 30 d[60]
Left main disease	No significant difference in the 2-y MACE rate compared with non–left main disease[49]	Low rates of periprocedural complications. At 1 y, the MACCE rate was 11.3% driven by MI[61,62]
Small vessels (≤2.5 mm)	Comparable 3-y clinical outcomes compared with the larger diameter group with similar rates of angiographic complications[51]	Small-diameter vessels seem to be feasible and safe at 30-d follow-up with similar rates of angiographic complications compared with the larger diameter group[63]
Long lesions (stent length of ≥50 mm)	-	Despite higher angiographic complication rates, similar 1-y event rates compared with lesions <50 mm[50]

Abbreviations: CABG, coronary artery bypass graft; MI, myocardial infarction.

The ViperWire tip should remain a minimum of 10 mm distal to the atherectomy burr during treatment. During ablation, the crown can move forward, and care should be taken to ensure adequate wire distance is maintained distal to the burr. If the burr advances too far distal, wire fracture is possible. Snare devices may be necessary for retrieving fractured wire tips.

Future Directions

The ongoing Evaluation of Treatment Strategies for Severe CaLcIfic Coronary Arteries: Orbital

OCT-guided approach to lesion preparation with orbital atherectomy

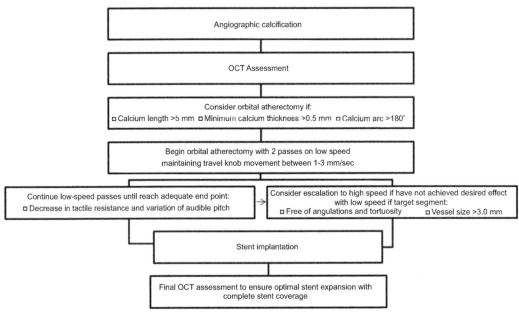

Fig. 2. Algorithm for an OCT-guided approach to lesion preparation with orbital atherectomy.

Atherectomy vs. Conventional Angioplasty Technique Prior to Implantation of Drug-Eluting StEnts: ECLIPSE trial (NCT03108456) is a landmark multicenter trial randomizing approximately 2000 patients with severely calcified lesions to either orbital atherectomy or balloon angioplasty before stent implantation. The primary endpoint of the study is target vessel failure, defined as the composite of cardiac death, target vessel–related MI, or

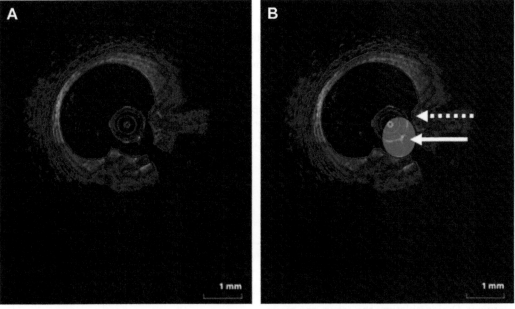

Fig. 3. (A) OCT cross-section image demonstrating the mechanism of action of OA with polishing of the calcified surface, with characteristic smooth, concave ablation and calcium fracture. (B) Dashed arrow indicating calcium fracture. Blue circle indicates region that was ablated, with wire visible (solid arrow). It is common for OA to treat the segment, where the OCT catheter and wire are visualized on the OCT cross-section.

ischemia-driven TVR. In addition, there is an OCT imaging subgroup cohort in which the primary endpoint will compare final minimal stent area between groups. The ECLIPSE trial is actively enrolling, and the final results are not expected until 2022. This will be the largest trial to date assessing PCI in severely calcified lesions.

SUMMARY

Detection and assessment of coronary calcification before PCI is essential to determine if lesion preparation is needed. Orbital atherectomy plays an important role in lesion preparation of calcified lesions before stent implantation to ensure optimal results by facilitating adequate stent expansion.

REFERENCES

1. Grüntzig AR, Senning Å, Siegenthaler WE. Nonoperative dilatation of coronary-artery stenosis: percutaneous transluminal coronary angioplasty. N Engl J Med 1979;301:61–8.
2. Madhavan MV, Tarigopula M, Mintz GS, et al. Coronary artery calcification: pathogenesis and prognostic implications. J Am Coll Cardiol 2014;63: 1703–14.
3. Kobayashi Y, Okura H, Kume T, et al. Impact of target lesion coronary calcification on stent expansion. Circ J 2014;78(9):2209–14.
4. Genereux P, Madhavan MV, Mintz GS, et al. Ischemic outcomes after coronary intervention of calcified vessels in acute coronary syndromes: pooled analysis from the HORIZONS-AMI (harmonizing outcomes with revascularization and stents in acute myocardial infarction) and ACUITY (acute catheterization and urgent intervention triage strategy) trials. J Am Coll Cardiol 2014;63:1845–54.
5. Mosseri M, Satler LF, Pichard AD, et al. Impact of vessel calcification on outcomes after coronary stenting. Cardiovasc Revasc Med 2005;6:147–53.
6. Lee MS, Shah N. The impact and pathophysiologic consequences of coronary artery calcium deposition in percutaneous coronary interventions. J Invasive Cardiol 2016;28:160–7.
7. Fujii K, Mintz GS, Kobayashi Y, et al. Contribution of stent underexpansion to recurrence after siromuseluting stent implantation for in-stent restenosis. Circulation 2004;109(9):1085–8.
8. Fujii K, Carlier SG, Mintz GS, et al. Stent underexpansion and residual reference segment stenosis are related to stent thrombosis after sirolimus-eluting stent implantation: an intravascular ultrasound study. J Am Coll Cardiol 2005;45(7):995–8.
9. Sonoda S, Morino Y, Ako J, et al. Impact of final stent dimensions on long-term results following sirolimus-eluting stent implantation: serial intravascular ultrasound analysis from the sirius trial. J Am Coll Cardiol 2004;43(11):1959–63.
10. Mintz GS, Popma JJ, Pichard AD, et al. Patterns of calcification in coronary artery disease. A statistical analysis of intravascular ultrasound and coronary angiography in 1155 lesions. Circulation 1995; 91(7):1959–65.
11. Wang X, Matsumura M, Mintz GS, et al. In vivo calcium detection by comparing optical coherence tomography, intravascular ultrasound, and angiography. JACC Cardiovasc Imaging 2017; 10(8):869–79.
12. Arora S, Panaich SS, Patel N, et al. Coronary atherectomy in the United States (from a Nationwide Inpatient Sample). Am J Cardiol 2016;117(4):555–62.
13. Armstrong EJ, Stanislawski MA, Kokkinidis DG, et al. Coronary atherectomy is associated with improved procedural and clinical outcomes among patients with calcified coronary lesions: insights from the VA CART program. Catheter Cardiovasc Interv 2018;91(6):1009–17.
14. Levine GN, Bates ER, Blankenship JC, et al, American College of Cardiology Foundation, American Heart Association Task Force on Practice Guidelines, Society for Cardiovascular Angiography and Interventions. 2011 ACCF/AHA/SCAI guideline for percutaneous coronary intervention: a report of the American College of Cardiology Foundation/American Heart Association Task Force on Practice Guidelines and the Society for Cardiovascular Angiography and Interventions. Catheter Cardiovasc Interv 2013;82(4):E266–355.
15. Barbato E, Shlofmitz E, Milkas A, et al. State of the art: evolving concepts in the treatment of heavily calcified and undilatable coronary stenoses - from debulking to plaque modification, a 40-year-long journey. EuroIntervention 2017;13(6):696–705.
16. Lee MS, Martinsen BJ, Shlofmitz R, et al. Coronary orbital atherectomy. In: Lanzer P, editor. Catheter-based cardiovascular interventions: a knowledge-based approach. 2nd edition. Cham (Switzerland): Springer Science & Business Media; 2018. p. 681–98.
17. Lee MS, Nguyen H, Philipson D, et al. "Single-operator" technique for advancing the orbital atherectomy device. J Invasive Cardiol 2017;29(3):92–5.
18. Shlofmitz E, Martinsen BJ, Lee M, et al. Orbital atherectomy for the treatment of severely calcified coronary lesions: evidence, technique, and best practices. Expert Rev Med Devices 2017;14(11): 867–79.
19. Sotomi Y, Shlofmitz R, Colombo A, et al. Patient selection and procedural considerations for coronary orbital atherectomy system. Interv Cardiol 2016;11(1):33–8.
20. Chambers JW, Diage T. Evaluation of the Diamondback 360 coronary orbital atherectomy

system for treating de novo, severely calcified lesions. Expert Rev Med Devices 2014;11:457–66.

21. Lee MS, Nguyen H, Shlofmitz R. Incidence of bradycardia and outcomes of patients who underwent orbital atherectomy without a temporary pacemaker. J Invasive Cardiol 2017;29(2):59–62.

22. Sotomi Y, Cavalcante R, Shlofmitz RA, et al. Quantification by optical coherence tomography imaging of the ablation volume obtained with the Orbital Atherectomy System in calcified coronary lesions. EuroIntervention 2016;12(9):1126–34.

23. Karimi Galougahi K, Shlofmitz RA, Ben-Yehuda O, et al. Guiding light: insights into atherectomy by optical coherence tomography. JACC Cardiovasc Interv 2016;9(22):2362–3.

24. Sharma S, Saito S, Shlofmitz R, et al. LBT-3 treatment of severely calcified coronary lesions with the coronary orbital atherectomy system micro crown: 1-year results from the COAST trial. JACC Cardiovasc Interv 2017;3(10):S1–2.

25. Maejima N, Hibi K, Saka K, et al. Relationship between thickness of calcium on optical coherence tomography and crack formation after balloon dilatation in calcified plaque requiring rotational atherectomy. Circ J 2016;80(6):1413–9.

26. Kubo T, Shimamura K, Ino Y, et al. Superficial calcium fracture after PCI as assessed by OCT. JACC Cardiovasc Imaging 2015;8(10):1228–9.

27. Fujino A, Mintz GS, Lee T, et al. Predictors of calcium fracture derived from balloon angioplasty and its effect on stent expansion assessed by optical coherence tomography. JACC Cardiovasc Interv 2018;11(10):1015–7.

28. Fujino A, Mintz GS, Matsumura M, et al. A new optical coherence tomography-based calcium scoring system to predict stent underexpansion. EuroIntervention 2018;13(18):e2182–9.

29. Parikh K, Chandra P, Choksi N, et al. Safety and feasibility of orbital atherectomy for the treatment of calcified coronary lesions: the ORBIT I trial. Catheter Cardiovasc Interv 2013;81(7):1134–9.

30. Bhatt P, Parikh P, Patel A, et al. Orbital atherectomy system in treating calcified coronary lesions: 3-year follow-up in first human use study (ORBIT I trial). Cardiovasc Revasc Med 2014;15(4):204–8.

31. Lee M, Généreux P, Shlofmitz R. Orbital atherectomy for treating de novo, severely calcified coronary lesions: 3-year results of the pivotal ORBIT II trial. Cardiovasc Revasc Med 2017;18(4):261–4.

32. Généreux P, Lee AC, Kim CY, et al. Orbital atherectomy for treating de novo severely calcified coronary narrowing (1-year results from the pivotal ORBIT II trial). Am J Cardiol 2015;115(12):1685–90.

33. Lee MS, Shlofmitz E, Kaplan B, et al. Real-world multicenter registry of patients with severe coronary artery calcification undergoing orbital atherectomy. J Interv Cardiol 2016;29(4):357–62.

34. Lee MS, Shlofmitz E, Goldberg A, et al. Multicenter registry of real-world patients with severely calcified coronary lesions undergoing orbital atherectomy: 1-year outcomes. J Invasive Cardiol 2018; 30(4):121–4.

35. Chambers JW, Feldman RL, Himmelstein SI, et al. Pivotal trial to evaluate the safety and efficacy of the orbital atherectomy system in treating de novo, severely calcified coronary lesions (ORBIT II). JACC Cardiovasc Interv 2014;7(5):510–8.

36. de Waha S, Allali A, Büttner HJ, et al. Rotational atherectomy before paclitaxel-eluting stent implantation in complex calcified coronary lesions: two-year clinical outcome of the randomized ROTAXUS trial. Catheter Cardiovasc Interv 2016;87(4): 691–700.

37. Yamamoto MH, Maehara A, Karimi Galougahi K, et al. Mechanisms of orbital versus rotational atherectomy plaque modification in severely calcified lesions assessed by optical coherence tomography. JACC Cardiovasc Interv 2017;10(24):2584–6.

38. Kini AS, Vengrenyuk Y, Pena J, et al. Optical coherence tomography assessment of the mechanistic effects of rotational and orbital atherectomy in severely calcified coronary lesions. Catheter Cardiovasc Interv 2015;86(6):1024–32.

39. Lee MS, Park KW, Shlofmitz E, et al. Comparison of rotational atherectomy versus orbital atherectomy for the treatment of heavily calcified coronary plaques. Am J Cardiol 2017;119(9):1320–3.

40. Okamoto N, Ueda H, Bhatheja S, et al. Procedural and one-year outcomes of patients treated with orbital and rotational atherectomy with mechanistic insights from optical coherence tomography. EuroIntervention 2018. [Epub ahead of print].

41. Meraj PM, Shlofmitz E, Kaplan B, et al. Clinical outcomes of atherectomy prior to percutaneous coronary intervention: a comparison of outcomes following rotational versus orbital atherectomy (COAP-PCI study). J Interv Cardiol 2018;31(4): 478–85.

42. Koifman E, Garcia-Garcia HM, Kuku KO, et al. Comparison of the efficacy and safety of orbital and rotational atherectomy in calcified narrowings in patients who underwent percutaneous coronary intervention. Am J Cardiol 2018;121(8):934–9.

43. Megaly M, Sandoval Y, Lillyblad MP, et al. Aminophylline for preventing bradyarrhythmias during orbital or rotational atherectomy of the right coronary artery. J Invasive Cardiol 2018;30(5):186–9.

44. Kim CY, Lee AC, Wiedenbeck TL, et al. Gender differences in acute and 30-day outcomes after orbital atherectomy treatment of de novo, severely calcified coronary lesions. Catheter Cardiovasc Interv 2016;87(4):671–7.

45. Lee MS, Shlofmitz E, Mansourian P, et al. Gender-based differences in outcomes after orbital

atherectomy for the treatment of de novo severely calcified coronary lesions. J Invasive Cardiol 2016; 28(11):440–3.

46. Lee MS, Shlofmitz RA, Martinsen BJ, et al. Impact of age following treatment of severely calcified coronary lesions with the orbital atherectomy system: 3-year follow-up. Cardiovasc Revasc Med 2018; 19(6):655–9.

47. Lee MS, Martinsen BJ, Lee AC, et al. Impact of diabetes mellitus on procedural and one year clinical outcomes following treatment of severely calcified coronary lesions with the orbital atherectomy system: a subanalysis of the ORBIT II study. Catheter Cardiovasc Interv 2018;91(6):1018–25.

48. Lee MS, Anose BM, Martinsen BJ, et al. Orbital atherectomy treatment of severely calcified native coronary lesions in patients with prior coronary artery bypass grafting: acute and one-year outcomes from the ORBIT II trial. Cardiovasc Revasc Med 2018;19(5 Pt A):498–502.

49. Lee MS, Shlofmitz E, Shlofmitz R, et al. Outcomes after orbital atherectomy of severely calcified left main lesions: analysis of the ORBIT II study. J Invasive Cardiol 2016;28(9):364–9.

50. Lee MS, Shlofmitz E, Lluri G, et al. One-year outcomes of orbital atherectomy of long, diffusely calcified coronary artery lesions. J Invasive Cardiol 2018;30(6):230–3.

51. Lee MS, Shlofmitz RA, Shlofmitz E, et al. Orbital atherectomy for the treatment of small (2.5mm) severely calcified coronary lesions: ORBIT II sub-analysis. Cardiovasc Revasc Med 2018;19(3 Pt A):268–72.

52. Lee MS, Shlofmitz E, Kong J, et al. Outcomes of patients with severely calcified aorto-ostial coronary lesions who underwent orbital atherectomy. J Interv Cardiol 2018;31(1):15–20.

53. Lee MS, Shlofmitz E, Nguyen H, et al. Outcomes in diabetic patients undergoing orbital atherectomy system. J Interv Cardiol 2016;29(5):491–5.

54. Whitbeck MG, Dewar J, Behrens AN, et al. Acute outcomes after coronary orbital atherectomy at a single center without on-site surgical backup: an experience in diabetics versus non-diabetics. Cardiovasc Revasc Med 2018;19(6S):12–5.

55. Lee MS, Shlofmitz E, Nayeri A, et al. Outcomes of patients with a history of coronary artery bypass grafting who underwent orbital atherectomy for severe coronary artery calcification. J Invasive Cardiol 2017;29(10):359–62.

56. Lee MS, Shlofmitz E, Lluri G, et al. Outcomes in elderly patients with severely calcified coronary lesions undergoing orbital atherectomy. J Interv Cardiol 2017;30(2):134–8.

57. Lee MS, Martinsen BJ, Shlofmitz R, et al. Orbital atherectomy treatment of severely calcified coronary lesions in patients with impaired left ventricular ejection fraction: one-year outcomes from the ORBIT II study. EuroIntervention 2017;13(3):329–37.

58. Shlofmitz E, Meraj P, Jauhar R, et al. Safety of orbital atherectomy in patients with left ventricular systolic dysfunction. J Interv Cardiol 2017;30(5): 415–20.

59. Lee MS, Lee AC, Shlofmitz RA, et al. ORBIT II subanalysis: impact of impaired renal function following treatment of severely calcified coronary lesions with the orbital atherectomy system. Catheter Cardiovasc Interv 2017;89(5):841–8.

60. Lee MS, Shlofmitz E, Lluri G, et al. Impact of impaired renal function in patients with severely calcified coronary lesions treated with orbital atherectomy. J Invasive Cardiol 2017;29(6):203–6.

61. Lee MS, Shlofmitz E, Kaplan B, et al. Percutaneous coronary intervention in severely calcified unprotected left main coronary artery disease: initial experience with orbital atherectomy. J Invasive Cardiol 2016;28(4):147–50.

62. Lee MS, Shlofmitz E, Park KW, et al. Orbital atherectomy of severely calcified unprotected left main coronary artery disease: one-year outcomes. J Invasive Cardiol 2018;30(7):270–4.

63. Lee MS, Shlofmitz E, Shlofmitz R. Outcomes of orbital atherectomy in severely calcified small (2.5 mm) coronary artery vessels. J Invasive Cardiol 2018;30(8):310–4.

64. Shlofmitz E, Martinsen B, Lee M, et al. Utilizing intravascular ultrasound imaging prior to treatment of severely calcified coronary lesions with orbital atherectomy: an ORBIT II sub-analysis. J Interv Cardiol 2017;30(6):570–6.

65. Shlofmitz E, Shlofmitz RA, Galougahi KK, et al. Algorithmic approach for optical coherence tomography-guided stent implantation during percutaneous coronary intervention. Interv Cardiol Clin 2018;7(3):329–44.

State-of-the-Art Coronary Artery Bypass Grafting

Patient Selection, Graft Selection, and Optimizing Outcomes

Mario F.L. Gaudino, MD, FEBCTS[a],*,
Cristiano Spadaccio, MD, PhD[b,c],
David P. Taggart, MD, PhD, FRCS[d,e]

KEYWORDS

- Coronary artery bypass grafting • Internal thoracic artery • Radial artery
- Hybrid revascularization • Percutaneous coronary intervention

---

KEY POINTS

- According to the most recent European Society of Cardiology guidelines on myocardial revascularization, patients with 3-vessel disease and Synergy between Percutaneous Coronary Intervention with TAXUS and Cardiac Surgery (SYNTAX) scores greater than 22, with or without concomitant diabetes mellitus, are best served by coronary artery bypass grafting (CABG).
- The left internal thoracic artery (ITA) is the conduit of choice and should be harvested in a skeletonized fashion to reduce the risk of sternal wound dehiscence.
- Multiarterial grafting improves mortality and event-free survival, and a multiple arterial grafting strategy should be the preferred approach in most patients undergoing CABG.
- The radial artery (RA) and right ITA should be used for conduits to the anterolateral wall. The RA is preferred for vessels with subocclusive target stenoses and patients at risk for sternal complications. The right ITA is preferred in patients without ulnar compensation. A saphenous vein graft should be considered for inferior wall lesions when arterial conduit grafting is not feasible on clinical or technical grounds.
- Minimization of aortic manipulation is critical to avoid perioperative cerebrovascular events, and an anaortic technique using off-pump revascularization with only in situ ITA and composite (Y or T) grafts may provide optimal outcomes.
- The Hybrid Coronary Revascularization trial is a large randomized study that will compare multivessel percutaneous coronary intervention (PCI) to sternal-sparing, off-pump, isolated left ITA grafting to the left anterior descending (LAD) artery combined with PCI to at least 1 non-LAD target in patients with low SYNTAX scores.

Disclosure: The authors declare no commercial or financial conflicts of interest or funding sources.
[a] Department of Cardiothoracic Surgery, Weill Cornell Medicine, NewYork–Presbyterian Hospital, 525 East 68th Street, New York, NY 10021, USA; [b] Department of Cardiothoracic Surgery, Golden Jubilee National Hospital, Agamemnon Street, Clydebank, Glasgow G81 4DY, UK; [c] University of Glasgow, Institute of Cardiovascular and Medical Sciences, 126 University Place, Glasgow G128TA, UK; [d] Department of Cardiovascular Surgery, University of Oxford, Headley Way, Oxford, Oxforshire OX39DU, UK; [e] Department Cardiac Surgery, John Radcliffe Hospital, Headley Way, Headington, Oxford, Oxfordshire OX3 9DU, UK
* Corresponding author.
E-mail address: mfg9004@med.cornell.edu

Intervent Cardiol Clin 8 (2019) 173–198
https://doi.org/10.1016/j.iccl.2018.11.007
2211-7458/19/© 2018 Elsevier Inc. All rights reserved.

INTRODUCTION

Coronary artery disease (CAD) remains a leading cause of death in Western countries. Treatment modalities for CAD include percutaneous coronary intervention (PCI) and coronary artery bypass grafting (CABG). The selection between these 2 approaches depends on several factors, including coronary anatomy, clinical presentation, and comorbidities. To date, several clinical trials and research efforts have been undertaken with the aim to provide data to identify the best approach to be adopted. Despite achieving some definitive evidence regarding the superiority of either modality, some subgroups of patients still remain in a gray zone and the indication for either approach remains borderline.[1,2]

Notwithstanding the progressive expansion of clinical indications for PCI and the associated technical advances in stent design, CABG remains the mainstay in patients with multivessel disease (MVD).[3,4] Despite an increasingly higher risk patient profile, improvement in surgical techniques and refinement of patient selection have resulted in improved outcomes for CABG, with reduced rates of operative mortality and major morbidity.[2,5,6] Large multicenter randomized and observational studies have reported excellent short-term outcomes,[7,8] whereas 5-year and 10-year survival rates are approximately equal to 85% to 95% and 75%, respectively.[2,9,10] Several technical advances could further optimize short-term and long-term outcomes after CABG, including developments in off-pump and no-touch procedures, total arterial revascularization with a careful conduit selection (including bilateral internal mammary artery and radial artery [RA] use), minimally invasive approaches, and more attentive postoperative management and surgical follow-up encouraging the compliance to medical treatment.[11] This article focuses on the latest advancements in indications, patient selection, practice patterns, and outcomes of CABG. Also, the contemporary strategies in use and under development to optimize CABG results are discussed.

INDICATIONS, PATIENT SELECTION, AND DECISION-MAKING CRITERIA

The main indications for myocardial revascularization, either with PCI or CABG, are to relieve anginal symptoms despite medical treatment and/or to improve survival. In this context, the revascularization strategy can be tailored according to the underlying pathologic mechanism (ie, stable CAD or acute coronary syndrome [ACS], including unstable angina with ST-segment elevation myocardial infarction [STEMI] or non-STEMI [NSTEMI]) and the anatomic and functional extent of the disease. However, several other factors interplay in the decision-making process, including the clinical presentation, comorbidities, cognitive status, estimated life expectancy, and the features of the specific revascularization modality. The heart team should consider individual cardiac and extracardiac characteristics, in addition to patient preference.[4] The most important criteria with respect to the type of revascularization to be adopted (CABG or PCI)[4] are the predicted surgical mortality relative to the patient's individual characteristics, the anatomic complexity of CAD that is present, and the anticipated completeness of revascularization (see later discussion).

Risk Evaluation

The recent European Society of Cardiology (ESC) guidelines on myocardial revascularization outline a detailed algorithm for risk stratification. Patients can be classified into 3 broad categories: very-high-risk, high-risk, and intermediate-risk. These categories mainly drive the timing for intervention, especially in the context of ACS.[4]

Predicted mortality for CABG can be estimated using EuroSCORE II (European System for Cardiac Operative Risk Evaluation)[12] and the Society of Thoracic Surgeons' risk model.[13] The latter scoring system also provides a calculated risk of stroke, renal failure, sternal wound infection, and length of stay.[13] The predictive ability of these 2 models performs equally in the setting of isolated CABG.[14] However, other comorbidities, such as pulmonary hypertension, liver disease, previous chest radiation, and the frailty status of the patient, should be included as significantly increasing the surgical risk.[15]

A summary of the cardiac and noncardiac variables to be assessed in the workup of CAD patients is listed in Table 1. In addition to the main comorbidities, the concomitant presence of noncoronary cardiac abnormalities (eg, valve disease, endocarditis, aortic involvement) deserves full attention because they are crucial determinants in the choice between PCI or CABG, and they significantly affect the operative planning and overall outcomes of surgery. Similarly, the hemodynamic status of the patient and the clinical urgency for surgery need to be considered to select the best timing for intervention. In this context, an appropriate diagnostic workup of patients before intervention is required and should include a full set of investigations such as clinical history, electrocardiogram, angiogram

Table 1
Workup for coronary artery disease patients

Variable	Details/History	Investigation
Demographic variables	Age, Sex	Clinical history
Previous cardiovascular events	Previous cardiovascular surgery Previous percutaneous intervention Previous myocardial infarction Previous stroke or Transient ischemic attack	Clinical history Carotid ultrasound
Disease complexity and disease	Number of disease vessels and extent of disease Concomitant valve or aorta disease Presence of endocarditis	Angiogram, SYNTAX score, FFR Transesophageal echocardiogram
Hemodynamic or clinical status	Urgent surgery required (NSTEMI, left main, ongoing symptoms)	Clinical evaluation
Cardiovascular variables	Diabetes mellitus Hypertension and cardiovascular risk factors Left ventricular function Previous or concurrent arrhythmias peripheral vascular disease	Clinical history Transthoracic echocardiogram Electrocardiogram, 24-h Holter
Noncardiovascular variables	Renal failure Chronic obstructive pulmonary disease	Blood test Pulmonary function tests

with the score evaluation from the Synergy Between Percutaneous Coronary Intervention With TAXUS (Paclitaxel-eluting stent, Boston Scientific, USA) and Cardiac Surgery (SYNTAX) trial, and fractional flow reserve (FFR) measurements, alongside carotid ultrasound in cases of diabetic patients, left main disease, previous cerebrovascular events, or clinical findings of carotid stenosis (Fig. 1; see Table 1).

Disease complexity

The assessment of the degree and complexity of coronary disease relies on both anatomic and functional parameters and recent guidelines emphasize the importance of SYNTAX score and FFR, respectively.[4] The SYNTAX score allows for a quantification of the degree of anatomic complexity by means of angiographic analysis of the location and length of lesions, of the presence of severe calcification, site of bifurcation or trifurcation (Medina score), presence of a chronic total occlusion or diffuse disease of small vessels, bifurcation or trifurcation lesions, and vessel tortuosity. Interestingly, although this score has been demonstrated to be prognostic predictor after PCI, it does not affect short-term and long-term outcomes in CABG,

thus constituting a solid factor to discriminate candidates for CABG instead of PCI.[4,16,17] In the latest ESC guidelines on myocardial revascularization, the original categorizations of low, intermediate, and high complexity has been synthesized and now combines the intermediate-risk and high-risk anatomy (SYNTAX score >22) as the group best served by CABG.[4]

FFR represents an emerging field of discussion, especially after the results of the Fractional Flow Reserve vs Angiography for Multivessel Evaluation (FAME)-2 study. This trial demonstrated that percutaneous revascularization of physiologically significant lesions defined by FFR improved the primary endpoint of death, nonfatal MI, or urgent revascularization within 2 years compared with medical treatment alone,[18] and this advantage was maintained over medical therapy at 3 years.[19] The functional investigation of vessel stenosis allows compensation for biases related to the subjective evaluation of anatomic parameters on the angiogram and can quantify the hemodynamic significance of a coronary lesion in terms of pressure drop across a stenosis. Studies have identified a cutoff of less than or equal to 0.80[20] to mandate intervention in PCI.[21] However, this concept is

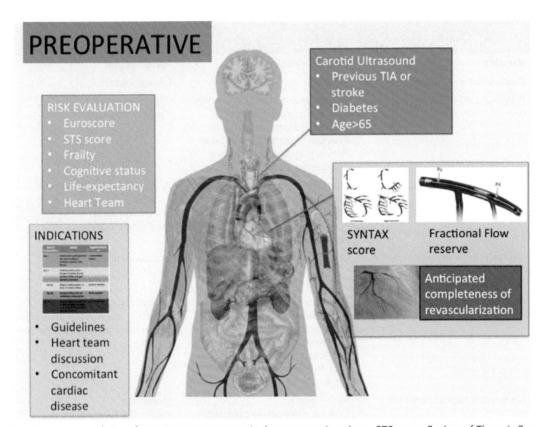

PREOPERATIVE

RISK EVALUATION
- Euroscore
- STS score
- Frailty
- Cognitive status
- Life-expectancy
- Heart Team

Carotid Ultrasound
- Previous TIA or stroke
- Diabetes
- Age>65

INDICATIONS

- Guidelines
- Heart team discussion
- Concomitant cardiac disease

SYNTAX score

Fractional Flow reserve

Anticipated completeness of revascularization

Fig. 1. Recommendations for patient management in the preoperative phase. STS score, Society of Thoracic Surgery (STS) score; TIA, transient ischemic attack.

also acquiring an important significance in the context of CABG, in light of early studies demonstrating that angiography-based assessment poorly correlates with the number of functionally significant lesions in individuals with MVD, and that this might lead to potentially unnecessary grafts.[22] Grafts of nonsignificant lesions have a higher rate of occlusion at 1 year[23] and accelerate atherosclerosis in native vessels, particularly when a venous graft is used.[24] For this reason, initial efforts investigating the role of FFR-guided CABG have been undertaken. Toth and colleagues[25] reported a reduced number of anastomoses and a higher rate of off-pump procedures with rates of major outcomes, composite of death, myocardial infarction (MI), and target vessel revascularization at 3-year follow-up comparable with standard CABG.

Anticipated Completeness of Revascularization

As demonstrated by the Clinical Outcomes Utilizing Revascularization and Aggressive Drug Evaluation (COURAGE) trial, the main aim of myocardial revascularization is to minimize residual ischemia.[26] It has been shown that a residual SYNTAX score greater than 8 after PCI significantly increases the 5-year risk of death and of the composite of death, MI, and stroke; and that any residual SYNTAX score greater than 0 is associated with the risk of repeat intervention.[26] A large meta-analysis, including 89,883 subjects enrolled in randomized clinical trials and observational studies confirmed better long-terms outcomes in terms of mortality and major cardiovascular events when an anatomic complete revascularization was achieved compared with an incomplete group.[27] Similar findings were derived from post hoc analysis of the SYNTAX trial, in which incomplete revascularization (IR) was associated with inferior long-term outcomes after both CABG and PCI.[28] A pooled analysis of the SYNTAX, Randomized Comparison of Coronary Artery Bypass Surgery and Everolimus-Eluting Stent Implantation in the Treatment of Patients With Multivessel Coronary Artery Disease (BEST), and Premier of Randomized Comparison of Bypass Surgery vs Angioplasty Using Sirolimus-Eluting Stent in Patients with Left Main Coronary Artery Disease (PRECOMBAT) trials demonstrated that PCI outcomes were comparable with CABG only when complete revascularization was achieved.[29] In a 5-year analysis of causes of death and cardiovascular events in the SYNTAX trial, IR was an independent predictor of mortality only in the PCI group, whereas in the CABG arm of the study IR did not increase the risk of death or cardiac adverse events, suggesting that surgical revascularization per se, despite its incompleteness, could protect patients from adverse events.[30] The positive effect of revascularization of left anterior descending artery (LAD) with the left internal thoracic artery (LITA) grafts has been proposed as an explanation of these findings.[31] Recently, a comprehensive meta-analysis has confirmed that, in the presence of a LITA-LAD graft, the impact of IR on survival is marginal when only 1 coronary territory is left ungrafted. However, the survival rate is significantly reduced if both the right coronary artery and circumflex territories are left ungrafted. IR in the context of off-pump CABG was associated with significantly lower survival even when only 1 coronary territory was not revascularized.[32] Therefore, the ability to achieve completeness of revascularization is a crucial question in when deciding whether to perform CABG and PCI in the setting of MVD.

Indications

Evidence from several randomized clinical trials and meta-analyses have delineated the subgroups of patients that mainly benefit from surgery or PCI (**Tables 2 and 3**). Initial analyses of the SYNTAX trial demonstrated an advantage with CABG in patients with intermediate or high anatomic complexity (as defined by SYNTAX score).[33,34] This benefit has been attributed to the placement of bypass grafts to the mid coronary vessels, which is thought to provide protection from the development of new proximal disease. The most recent and comprehensive subject-level meta-analysis, including data from all the currently available randomized trials (both on multivessel and left main disease), reported a significant survival benefit with CABG over PCI at 5-year follow-up (all-cause mortality 11.2% after PCI and 9.2% after CABG; hazard ratio 1.20, 95% CI 1.06–1.37, P = .0038), suggesting diabetes and the high complexity of coronary disease as outcome-modifier variables.[9] A large subject-level meta-analysis, combining the results of the SYNTAX and BEST trials, confirmed improved outcomes in CABG when compared with drug-eluting stent-PCI, regardless of the diabetes status, as well as in MVD (2 or 3 vessels involved) with proximal LAD involvement.[35] Another analysis by Chang and colleagues[36] demonstrated similar benefit in nondiabetic

patients with intermediate-to-high SYNTAX scores. Another factor marking a significant watershed in the indications for CABG is represented by poor left ventricular (LV) function, as demonstrated by the Surgical Treatment for Ischemic Heart Failure (STICH) trial.[37,38]

In the context of left main disease, the available evidence is represented by the Everolimus-Eluting Stents or Bypass Surgery for Left Main Coronary Artery Disease (EXCEL)[39] and the Nordic-Baltic-British Left Main Revascularization Study (NOBLE)[40] trials. A pooled analysis showed equivalence of PCI and CABG with respect to clinical outcomes in low-to-intermediate complexity SYNTAX scores. However, PCI benefit was offset by a higher risk of spontaneous MI during long-term follow-up and by a significant higher need for repeat revascularization when compared with CABG.[41] The pooled analysis of randomized trials by Head and colleagues[9] showed similar outcomes for the subgroup of left main disease in the PCI and CABG groups regardless of other variables. However, the results of these studies have been recently questioned because of methodological flaws and insufficient power to perform a valid subgroup analysis, therefore impeding drawing any reliable conclusions regarding the various subcategories of patients identified.[42]

Based on this evidence, and on the previously mentioned parameters and decision-making criteria, the recent ESC guidelines recommend CABG in proximal LAD single vessel and double vessel disease, triple vessel disease with intermediate-risk or high-risk SYNTAX score in nondiabetic patients, and in triple vessel disease in diabetic patients independent of the SYNTAX complexity. Similarly, left main disease in intermediate-risk or high-risk SYNTAX is an indication for CABG, whereas the option of PCI as an alternative is available in low-risk SYNTAX.[4] However, further evidence is required to demonstrate the actual equivalence of the 2 treatments.[42] Diabetes, poor LV function, diffuse calcific disease with previous episodes of intrastent restenosis, predicted inability to achieve complete revascularization in lower SYNTAX score, contraindications to dual antiplatelet therapy, and concomitant valve or aortic surgery are additional factors favoring the choice of CABG. Conversely, major technical contraindications to surgery, frailty, comorbidities not considered in the available models associated with high risk, porcelain aorta, or lack of conduits should lead to consideration of PCI (**Table 4**). **Fig. 1** summarizes the recommendations in the preoperative phase of surgical patient management.

Table 2
Overview of randomized controlled trials: percutaneous coronary intervention versus coronary artery bypass grafting

Study (Year of Publication)	Country	Inclusion Criteria	SYNTAX Score Mean (≥33)	Number of Vessels Diseased	Number of Subjects Assigned CABG	DES-PCI	Medically Treated Diabetes (on Insulin)	Stents Used	Median Follow-up (y)	Notes
CARDia,[193] 2010	United Kingdom and Ireland	Diabetics with MVD, including PLAD	NR	3VD: 63% 2VD: 32% PLAD: 5%	242	248	100% (38%)	SES (69%) BMS (31%)	1	PCI might be feasible in diabetic with MDV
FREEDOM,[194] 2012	Multinational	Diabetes and stenosis of >70% in ≥2 major epicardial vessels	26 (19%)	3VD: 83% 2VD: 17%	947	953	100% (32%)	SES (51%) PES (43%)	3.8	CABG superior to PCI for mortality MI but higher stroke risk
VA CARDS,[195] 2013	United States	Diabetics with MVD, including PLAD	22 (13%)	3VD: 63% 2VD: 24% PLAD: 13%	97	101	100% (47%)	SES (20%) PES (35%) EES (18%) ZES (2%) Mixed (16%) BMS (1%)	2	CABG superior to PCI but enrollment stopped prematurely
SYNTAX,[33] 2014	Multinational	Significant stenosis in vessels supplying all 3 major epicardial territories	28, NR	3VD: 100% 2VD: 0%	549	546	27% (11%)	PES	5	CABG superior to PCI, lower rates of death, MI, and repeat revascularization, stroke rate similar
BEST trial,[196] 2015	South Korea, China, Malaysia, and Thailand	Stenoses of >70% of the vessel diameter in major epicardial vessels in the territories of at least 2 coronary arteries	24 (16%)	3VD: 77% 2VD: 23%	442	438	41% (4%)	EES	2	CABG superior to PCI, lower rate of MACCE
PRECOMBAT,[197] 2015	Korea	Unprotected left main disease	Mean 25	LMCA	300	300	30%	SES	5	No difference in MACCE rate
EXCEL,[39] 2016	Multinational	LMCA	≤32	LMCA	957	948	30%	EES	3	PCI noninferior to CABG for composite endpoint of death, stroke, MI
NOBLE,[40] 2016	Multinational (36 centers)	Left main disease	Mean 22.5	LMCA	603	598	15%	SES PES	5	CABG better than PCI (mortality, MI, repeat revascularization stroke)

Abbreviations: 2VD, 2-vessel disease; 3VD, 3-vessel disease; BMS, bare-metal stent; CARDia, The Coronary Artery Revascularisation in Diabetes trial; DES, drug-eluting stent; EES, everolimus eluting stent; EXCEL, Everolimus-Eluting Stents or Bypass Surgery for Left Main Coronary Artery Disease; FREEDOM, The Future REvascularization Evaluation in patients with Diabetes mellitus: optimal management of Multivessel disease trial; LMCA, left main coronary artery; MACCE, major adverse cardiac and cerebrovascular events; VA CARDS, Coronary Artery Revascularization in Diabetes (Veterans Affairs); NOBLE, Nordic-Baltic-British Left Main Revascularization Study; NR, not reported; PES, paclitaxel-eluting stent; PLAD, proximal LAD; SES, sirolimus-eluting stent; SYNTAX, Synergy Between Percutaneous Coronary Intervention With TAXUS and Cardiac Surgery; ZES, zotarolimus-eluting stent.

Table 3
Overview of meta-analyses of studies comparing percutaneous coronary intervention with coronary artery bypass grafting

Author, Date	Studies Included	Total Number of Subjects	Years at Follow-up	Mortality	Stroke or Cerebrovascular Event	MI	Repeat Revascularization (RR)	Notes
Hakeem et al,[198] 2013	4 RCTs	3052	4 y	Favors CABG	Favors PCI	Favors CABG	Favors CABG	CABG in diabetic patients with MVD at low to intermediate surgical risk (EuroSCORE <5) is superior to MVD PCI with DES
Garcia et al,[27] 2013	35 studies	89,883	—	—	—	—	—	CR is more commonly achieved with CABG than PCI. IR has increased mortality and RR independently of the mode of treatment
Al Ali et al,[199] 2014	7 RCTs MVD + LMD	5835	6 m–5 y	Favors CABG	Favors PCI	Favors CABG	Favors CABG	In MVD patients, CABG reduced the risk of mortality but increased stroke risk. In subjects with LMD, CABG reduced revascularization risk and increased stroke risk
Sipahi et al,[200] 2014	6 RCTs	6055	4.1 y	Favors CABG	Nonsignificant	Favors CABG	Favors CABG	CABG is superior to PCI independently of diabetes
Lim et al,[201] 2014	5 RCTs; 9 OBS	5000	3–5 y	Favors CABG	30 d: favors PCI 1y–5y: Nonsignificant	Favors CABG	Favors CABG	Cardiovascular or cerebrovascular events were 1.71 times higher in the DES-PCI
D'Ascenzo et al,[202] 2014	20 RCTs aimed at correlating risk factors	12,844	30 d–1 y	Favors CABG	Favors PCI	Favors CABG	Favors CABG	PCI reduces the risk of stroke in women; PCI has increased risk of RR risk in women and in those with diabetes
Fanari et al,[203] 2015	6 RCTs	5123	1 y + 5 y	1 y: nonsignificant 5 y: favors CABG	Favors PCI	1 y: nonsignificant 5 y: favors CABG	Favors CABG	Increased death in diabetics with PCI

(continued on next page)

Table 5
(continued)

Author, Date	Studies Included	Total Number of Subjects	Years at Follow-up	Mortality	Stroke or Cerebrovascular Event	MI	Repeat Revascularization (RR)	Notes
Zimarino et al,[204] 2016	28 studies	83,695	4.7 ± 4.3 y	—	—	—	—	CR confers benefit on outcomes more evident in diabetics
Benedetto et al,[205] 2016	5 RCTs	4563	3–4 y	Favors CABG	Favors PCI	Favors CABG	Favors CABG	PCI increased mortality by 51% PCI increased MI by 102% CABG increased stroke by 29%
Lee et al,[206] 2016	3 RCTs MVD + LMD	3280	5 y	MVD: favors CABG LMD: nonsignificant	Nonsignificant	MVD: favors CABG LMD: favors CABG	Favors CABG	Overall CABG educed long-term rates of the composite of all-cause death, MI, or stroke in patients with LMD and MVD Benefit of CABG more pronounced in MVD
Chang et al,[36] 2016	BEST + SYNTAX in nondiabetics	1275	62 mo	Favors CABG	No differences	Favors CABG	Favors CABG	CABG compared with DES-PCI educed the long-term risk of mortality in nondiabetic patients with MVD CAD
Giacoppo et al,[41] 2017	4 RCTs LMD stenosis, PCI vs CABG, only of DES	4394	5 y	No differences	No differences	No differences	Favors CABG	Equivalence of mortality, stroke, MI PCI increased repeated revascularization Only LMD trial analyzed without MVD
Cavalcante et al,[35] 2017	BEST + SYNTAX	1166	5 y	Favors CABG	No differences	Favors CABG	Favors CABG	In MVD with proximal LAD involvement, CABG has lower rates of the composite endpoint of death, MI, or stroke.
Head et al,[9] 2018	11 RCTs MVD + LMD	11,518	5 y	Favors CABG in complex MVD and diabetes LMD: nonsignificant	—	—	—	CABG benefit restricted to MVD + diabetes Equivalence for LMD Equivalence for MVD in nondiabetic patients

Abbreviations: CR, complete revascularization; DES, drug-eluting stent; IR, incomplete revascularization; LMD, left main disease; OBS, observational; RCT, randomized controlled trial.

Table 4 Indications and factors considered by heart team in the choice between percutaneous coronary intervention and coronary artery bypass grafting	
Favors PCI	**Favors CABG**
MVD SYNTAX <22	MVD SYNTAX ≥23
Presence of severe comorbidities not reflected in current scoring systems	Diabetes
Advanced age, frailty, reduced life expectancy	Reduced LV function <35%
Severely restricted mobility impairing postoperative rehabilitation	Contraindications to DAPT
Severe chest deformation or scoliosis	Recurrent diffuse intrastent restenosis
Sequelae of chest radiation	Severely calcified coronary artery lesions limiting lesion expansion
Porcelain aorta	Indication for concomitant valve or ascending aorta surgery
Lack of conduits impeding complete revascularization with CABG	Predicted inability to achieve complete revascularization with PCI

Abbreviations: DAPT, dual anti-platelet therapy; LV, left ventricle.

CONDUIT SELECTION

Conduits available for CABG include the LITA grafts and the right internal thoracic artery (RITA) grafts, the RA, the right gastroepiploic artery (RGEA), and a saphenous vein (SV). The prognostic benefit of arterial grafts, especially LITA grafts on the left anterior descending, as well as their superiority over SV in terms of short-term and long-term outcomes has been widely accepted.[43,44] Several factors interplay in the choice of the grafting strategy for non-LAD targets in a particular patient's life expectancy, risk factors for sternal wound complications, coronary anatomy, degree of target vessel stenosis, graft quality, and surgical expertise. The characteristics of each conduit are discussed separately.

Internal Thoracic Artery

A large body of evidence supports the use of the internal thoracic arteries (ITAs), the LITA grafts in

particular, as the conduit of choice for CABG. Favorable histologic characteristics, as well as increased production of vasoactive molecules and antiinflammatory cytokines,[45] are thought to underlie the largely superior patency rate observed in this conduit compared with others. Other explanations for the superior outcomes reported for this conduit include the reduced tendency for spasm due to the lack of a significant muscle layer, and the relative protection from the development of atherosclerosis guaranteed by its biological properties.[46]

The LITA grafts can be harvested in a skeletonized or pedicled fashion. The former technique increases the effective length of the conduit available for grafting (normal length ranging from 14.32–19.48 cm)[47] and enables sequential anastomoses, if required. Avoidance of extensive devascularization of the sternum also has advantages in terms of minimizing complications with sternal wound healing. Skeletonization of the ITA has been reported to reduce the risk for deep sternal wound infections in diabetic patients, who are more prone to this complication,[48–50] and to provide higher blood flow compared with the pedicled technique.[51] For these reasons, skeletonization is also recommended by the current ESC guidelines.[4]

Long-term outcomes of LITA grafting show a greater than 90% patency rate at 20-year follow-up when it is used as a conduit to the LAD.[46,52] Similar patency rates were observed when the LITA grafts was anastomosed to the circumflex artery (patency of 97% at 5 years, 92% at 8 years, 89% at 10 years, and 91% at 15 years), whereas its patency was reduced to 84% at 15 years when it was used to graft the right coronary artery.[52] This discrepancy in performance between LITA grafts patency rates for the left and right systems is probably due vessel diameter mismatch and to the different rate of disease progression at the crux of the heart.[53] However, the results of the LITA grafts to either the left or right coronary system still outperforms the patency rate of an SV graft (SVG), which falls below 75% at 10-year follow-up.[54] The RITA grafts demonstrated a similar patency rate of around 90% to the left system and between 80% and 90% to the right system at 10-year follow-up. Histomorphological differences between the RITA grafts and the LITA grafts might explain this discrepancy in outcomes.[55]

In multiple meta-analyses, the use of bilateral ITA (BITA) grafts has been shown to significantly improve long-term survival compared with single ITA (SITA) grafts.[56] These findings have been repeatedly confirmed by large observational studies, which also demonstrated lower incidence of MI, recurrent angina, or reoperation with BITA grafting.[57–64] Subgroup analyses have shown that BITA use provide the greatest benefit for patients younger than 60 to 70 years of age.[65–67] Despite the apparent advantages of BITA grafting, there is reluctance among some cardiac surgeons to adopt this technique because of the perceived technical complexity and the concern for wound complications. In addition, a specific volume-outcome relationship has been recently identified.[68]

The Arterial Revascularization Trial (ART) was a randomized controlled trial designed to compare outcomes of SITA versus BITA revascularization in 3102 subjects undergoing CABG. At 5-year follow-up, there was no difference in the rates of death or the composite of death, MI, or stroke between treatment arms. There was a significantly increased risk of sternal wound dehiscence in the BITA group, especially in obese and diabetic patients.[69] In a post hoc, exploratory analysis that compared subjects who received 2 arterial grafts (BITA or LITA plus RA) with those who received only SITA, multiarterial grafting improved mortality and event-free survival. This risk of sternal dehiscence may be minimized by skeletonization of the ITAs.[70]

Several factors may explain the discordance between the results of ART and prior meta-analyses. A high crossover rate (14% of subjects did not undergo BITA despite allocation to that group), the frequent use of the RA in both groups, and a remarkable degree of compliance with medical treatment for secondary prevention may have diluted the benefit of BITA.[71–73] Indeed, a preliminary, as-treated analysis of the 10-year follow-up of the ART demonstrated a significant benefit with BITA revascularization (David P Taggart, EACTS [European Association of Cardithoracic Surgery] Meeting 2018, Milan, Italy, personal communication). The observed event rates were substantially lower than expected, resulting in substantial underpowering. The presence of unmatched and unmeasured confounders in the retrospective series, even if propensity-matched, might have led to treatment allocation bias.[74] The publication of subsequent data from a meta-analysis on BITA and from pooled analysis of the trials comparing the RA and the SV as a second graft, which demonstrated the superiority of total arterial-based CABG over SITA, strengthen the argument in favor of multiple arterial grafting. On the other hand, the present contradiction among studies raises the specter of hidden confounders and methodological flaws in the currently available literature and warrant the design of new randomized clinical trials to provide a definitive answer to the question of the potential clinical benefit of multiple arterial grafts. The results of the recently started Randomized Comparison of the Clinical Outcome of Single vs Multiple Arterial Grafts (ROMA; NCT03217006) trial, which will compare the impact of 1 ITA with 2 or more arterial grafts on the composite of death, stroke, postdischarge MI, and/or repeat revascularization in approximately 4300 subjects, are eagerly awaited.[75]

The Radial Artery

The RA was introduced as surgical conduit in the 1970s.[76] Its histologic peculiarities, featuring a well-developed muscular profile, fueled concerns of vasospasm after implantation. For this reason, calcium channel blockers with or without long-acting nitrates have been widely used in the postoperative period.[77] However, biological studies demonstrated a progressive remodeling toward a more elastomuscular phenotype after implantation as graft,[78] and clinical reports reported no benefit of spasmolytic pharmacologic therapy.[79] The use of this conduit has been progressively reintroduced since the early 1990s[80] and angiographic studies have demonstrated patency rates of 80% to 90% at 7 to 10 years follow-up.[81] A more recent study reported an 84.4% patency rate at 20 years with a probability of 20-year graft failure the same as a LITA grafts ($19.0 \pm 0.2\%$ for LITA grafts vs $25.0 \pm 0.2\%$ for the RA).[82] At least 6 randomized clinical trials and several observational studies have compared patency rates and outcomes of RA versus RITA grafts and SVG conduits, and recent evidence from a large patient-level meta-analysis has led to the renaissance of the RA conduit.[83] When compared with SVG, randomized trials and meta-analyses have shown a significantly higher patency rate and lower incidence of clinical events.[84–92] The most recent summary evidence from a patient-level meta-analysis comparing RA and SVG demonstrated a lower rate of adverse cardiac events and a higher rate of patency at 5 years of follow-up in the RA group.[83]

With respect to RITA grafts, the Radial Artery Patency and Clinical Outcomes (RAPCO) trial demonstrated no difference in the patency of the 2 conduits with a trend toward improved event-free survival in the RA group at the 6-year follow-up.[87] A meta-analysis of propensity-matched observational studies revealed that the skeletonized RITA grafts compared with RA was associated with superior long-term survival and freedom from repeat revascularization, with similar operative mortality and incidence of sternal wound complications.[93] Another pooled analysis of angiographic outcomes demonstrated a nonsignificant 27% absolute risk reduction for late functional graft failure in the RITA grafts compared with RA.[92] However, a meta-analysis, including both randomized controlled trials and observational studies, analyzing clinical outcomes demonstrated comparable mortality but reduced incidence of cardiac events in the RA group.[94] From a practical perspective, it has been suggested that RA might be a better option in patients at increased risk for postoperative sternal complications. Hoffman and colleagues[95] and Tranbaugh and colleagues,[96] in 2 separate propensity-matched studies, supported the benefits of RA in patients at risk of sternal complications, including the easily tolerable harvesting in frail patients and the avoidance of additional sternal devascularization.[94] In addition, a subanalysis of the Radial Artery Patency Study (RAPS) on diabetic subjects described a significant risk reduction on graft occlusion using RA,[84] making the use of this conduit in diabetics particularly attractive.

The RA can be harvested in a skeletonized or pedicled fashion and with an open or endoscopic technique. Although there may be an advantage in terms of conduit length and diameter if the RA is harvested in skeletonized fashion,[97] this approach is associated with a longer harvesting time and a risk for endothelial damage, especially when a harmonic scalpel is used.[98] Therefore, this approach should be discouraged given the lack of clear evidence of a significant improvement in patency rate using the skeletonization technique.[99] There is a paucity of evidence regarding the safety and efficacy of endoscopic harvesting,[100,101] and the success of the use of RA conduits in CABG does not seem to be influenced by an open incision or a minimally invasive endoscopic approach.

Conversely, the degree of coronary stenosis influences the long-term patency rate of RA grafts. A vessel stenosis greater than 70% is considered the only indication for RA grafting; a stenosis of greater than or equal to 90% is associated with even better results.[82,84] In a large angiographic study, target vessel location and the proximal and distal anastomosis sites did not significantly influence the patency rate at 6.5 years[102] and 20 years follow-up.[82] Given these promising results, research efforts have focused on whether the RA, rather than an SVG, might be a better adjunct to BITA use in CABG. Although a propensity-matched analysis with a mean follow-up of 10.6 years did not

show any difference in survival among subjects receiving an RA or SVG in addition to BITA,[103] a longer-term follow-up study demonstrated improved survival beyond 10-year follow-up in the RA group.[104] Furthermore, a propensity-matched analysis demonstrated a significant survival advantage at 15-year follow-up when RA was added to BITA grafting compared with SVG.[105] The survival benefit of a third arterial conduit, irrespective of sex and diabetic status, has been confirmed by 2 meta-analyses.[106,107]

Preoperatively, the anastomosis among the radial and ulnar system may be evaluated by the Allen test. A normal Allen test demonstrates sufficient collateralization of the 2 systems and, therefore, the functional compensation of the ulnar artery if the RA is harvested as a conduit for CABG. However, this test has been shown to be unreliable, and more objective methods to measure of ulnar compensation can be used, such as Doppler ultrasound and percutaneous oxymetry.[99,108] Importantly, considering the usual practice of performing preoperative angiography with radial access, the use of previously punctured RA is discouraged because of potential endothelial damage.[109,110]

The Right Gastroepiploic Artery

The RGEA (or right gastro-omental artery) is 1 of the 2 terminal branches of the gastroduodenal artery, running along the greater gastric curvature, between omental layers and eventually anastomosing with the left gastroepiploic artery from the splenic artery. From a histologic perspective, despite sharing the same wall thickness as ITA,[111] the RGEA contains several smooth muscle cells in the media, raising potential spasmogenic concerns during surgical manipulation.[112] Pym and colleagues[113] and Suma and colleagues[114] independently described the first use of the RGEA in CABG in 1987. In early hemodynamic studies, Takayama and colleagues[115] demonstrated that harvested RGEA maintained its physiologic behavior after exercise or digestion and featured good flow capacity after endothelial stimulation with vasoactive substances.[116] Also, it was burdened by a very low incidence of severe atherosclerosis.[117]

In clinical settings, RGEA is readily available and large angiographic studies on anatomic length and diameter of the conduit demonstrated 97% and 88% probability to reach right coronary and circumflex artery, respectively. Only a few contraindications to RGEA use were described in an early study by Saito and colleagues,[118] permitting to assume availability of RGEA for every case without the need for a preoperative angiographic evaluation. Similarly, no increase in perioperative risk was identified when compared with subjects in whom the RGEA was not used.[119]

The most favorable target for the in situ right gastroepiploic artery (RGEA) graft is the distal right coronary artery, although the distal circumflex can also be grafted with this conduit. However, it is recommended to select a target vessel with a subocclusive (>90%) stenosis to maximize patency rates and avoid spasm or issues with competitive flow.[120] In a recent review of evidence and experience with RGEA over 30 years, Suma[112] described a 97% short-term patency rate and 90% patency rate at 10 years, especially when RGEA was harvested in a skeletonized fashion and anastomosed on target vessels with greater than 90% stenoses.[121] Although a network meta-analysis of randomized controlled trials reported a higher graft occlusion risk of RGEA compared with other conduits,[92] a large series described 5-year, 10-year, and 15-year actuarial survival rates of 91.7%, 81.4%, and 71.3%, respectively.[122] Moreover, superiority in terms of late survival with the use of RGEA instead of an SVG has been reported in 2 separate series.[123,124] Advocates of its use emphasize the importance of the skeletonized technique[121] and the selection of appropriate targets as reliable precautions to achieve success,[112] although most of the currently available literature focuses on the use of a pedicled RGEA. Currently, there are only few studies comparing RGEA with RITA grafts,[125,126] impeding a comprehensive picture in this context.

The Saphenous Vein

The greater SV (or long SV) is the most commonly used graft for CABG. From the biological and histologic point of view, several differences have been described in comparison with ITA, mainly regarding its intrinsic structure, a reduced production of endothelial nitric oxide, and an impaired secretory pattern of cytokines after implantation in the coronary system.[46,127–129] Since the initial study by Motwani and Topol,[127] the intrinsic morphologic and functional characteristics of the conduit and the harvesting technique have been considered the main factors responsible for the incidence of graft failure (both acute and chronic) and the disappointing long-term patency rates (75% at 18 months[130]). For this reason, a significant amount of experimental effort has been made with the aim to minimize trauma during harvesting or to enhance biological properties of the vein. Souza[131] described

the no-touch technique in 1996, in which the dissection of the SVG is performed leaving its surrounding tissue in situ. This technique is thought to prevent spasm related to adventitial denudation during harvesting, as well as to avoid smooth muscle cell activation,[132] and to preserve integrity of the vasa vasorum and endothelial function.[133] A recent randomized trial showed superiority of this technique over the standard harvesting in terms of long-term patency with rates comparable to ITA.[134] However, it has been suggested that the increased potential for wound infection and bleeding related to the greater invasiveness of the procedure might offset the advantage of this technique in terms of conduit integrity preservation and future patency rates.[135] The SVG can also be harvested endoscopically, with the benefit of avoiding a large leg incision with associated wound healing problems and pain, especially when the median saphenous nerve is accidentally damaged.[136,137] Initial concerns about the patency of SVG harvested endoscopically were raised in a post hoc analysis of the PREVENT (The Project of Ex-Vivo Vein Graft Engineering via Transfection) IV trial in which this technique was associated with vein-graft failure and adverse clinical outcomes.[138] Potential structural damage during harvesting likely explains these findings.[139] Although a meta-analysis supported these results,[140] there is not an unequivocal consensus regarding the inferiority of endoscopic SVG harvesting[137,141] and the results of a large angiographic study, the Randomized Endo-Vein Graft Prospective (REGROUP) trial, should potentially shed light on this question. Moreover, a subanalysis of the large Veterans Affairs Randomized On/Off Bypass (ROOBY) trial, showed a lower SVG patency rate in the off-pump group when harvested endoscopically.[142,143]

An interesting approach has been suggested by Kim and colleagues. The Saphenous Vein Versus Right Internal Thoracic Artery as a Y-Composite Graft (SAVE RITA) trial, compared the outcomes of SVG anastomosed as a Y-graft on the LITA grafts and used to graft both the left and right systems compared with the use of a RITA grafts.[144] The rationale underlying this method is that an SVG anastomosed to the LITA grafts may undergo reduced circulatory stress compared with an SVG anastomosed to the ascending aorta, and it would be continuously exposed to endothelium-protective substances, such as nitric oxide, produced by the LITA grafts.[145,146] Additionally, the avoidance of an aortic cross-clamp for creation of the proximal anastomosis might minimize the risk of stroke and aortic dissection. Sparing of the RITA grafts might also decrease the chances of sternal wound infection while preserving this conduit in case of the need for future redo cardiac surgery. At 1-year angiographic follow-up, the SV composite graft was noninferior to the RITA composite graft.[144] Five-years results have demonstrated similar findings; however, as recently reported, more evidence is needed to confirm the noninferiority of arteriovenous conduits for CABG.[147]

Another attractive approach to improve graft patency is to biologically augment the SVG to improve the resistance of this conduit to atherosclerosis and subsequent failure. The PREVENT IV trial investigated the role of ex vivo treatment with edifoligide, an E2F decoy that regulates expression of genes controlling smooth muscle cell proliferation and potentially prevents neointimal hyperplasia. However, this approach was ineffective in the prevention of early vein graft failure.[148] Another strategy entails the use of external stenting of SVG with the aim of preventing pressure-induced wall stress and reactive neointimal hyperplasia. Despite favorable preclinical data, the clinical results for this approach are conflicting to date.[149] An external venous nitinol-based mesh, the eSVS MESH (Kips Bay Medical, Minneapolis, MN, USA), did not produce encouraging results at 1 year (patency rate of reinforced SVG 76% vs nonreinforced SVG 100% and arterial grafts 100%).[150] Newer technologies, such as the VEST (Vascular Graft Solutions, Tel Aviv, Israel) device, which is a cobalt chromium external stent, have shown comparable patency to nonstented grafts[151] and significant improvements in hemodynamic flow within the stents.[152] Ongoing studies will determine whether this translates into superior graft patency over the longer term.

Grafting Strategy and Conduit Choice

When deciding on a grafting strategy, particular attention should be given to technical, anatomic, and angiographic determinants of arterial conduit patency, as well as the clinical characteristics of the patient (morbid characteristics, diabetes, obesity, respiratory problems, steroid, or immunosuppression treatments, especially if they occur simultaneously). According to guidelines, 1 ITA should always be anastomosed to the LAD, given the widely established prognostic benefit of this strategy. With respect to the second and following grafts, several combinations and constructions are available. These can be broadly grouped into a single or multiple arterial strategy. In the former, vein grafts are used for the remaining targets in the left and

right systems; in the latter, a second arterial conduit (ie, RITA, RA, or RGEA) can be used to graft the remaining targets on both the right and left side, or just on the left side, using an SVG on the right system. RA is recommended for targets bearing greater than 90% stenosis.

Based on the evidence currently available and given the long-term results of previous and new randomized clinical trials,[153] a multiple arterial grafting strategy should be the preferred approach in most patients. An ad hoc decisional algorithm has been recently suggested (**Fig. 2**).[154] In particular, the RA and RITA grafts should be used for conduits to the anterolateral wall, with the RA preferred in patients at risk for sternal complications and the RITA grafts in patients without ulnar compensation. The RA can be used in sequential anastomoses to reach every distal vessel; however, this conduit is recommended for subocclusive target stenoses because it is more sensitive to competitive coronary flow than the RITA grafts. The skeletonized in situ RGEA can be considered for grafting the distal branches of the right coronary artery when they are critically stenosed (>90%). An SVG is mainly considered for inferior wall lesions in the case that arterial conduit grafting is not feasible on clinical or technical grounds.

OPTIMIZING OUTCOMES

Outcome optimization in CABG is a multidimensional task requiring interventions or practice modifications at different levels in patient's care, including candidate selection (see **Fig. 1**), graft selection, intraoperative techniques (**Fig. 3**), and postoperative management (**Fig. 4**). Patient selection strategy and choice of conduits have been previously discussed. The following section focuses on the measures to optimize results in the intraoperative and postoperative management.

Intraoperative Management
Intraoperative quality control
Intraoperative graft assessment is recommended to check potential issues related to anastomotic imprecision, graft kinking, and limited graft outflow.

Transit-time flow measurement is among the most commonly adopted techniques and has shown that 2% to 4% of grafts can require revision.[155,156] Graft flow or pulsatility index are predictors of short-term complications, as well as death and graft failure during follow-up.[156] This technique is amenable to combination with epicardial echocardiography to provide both a

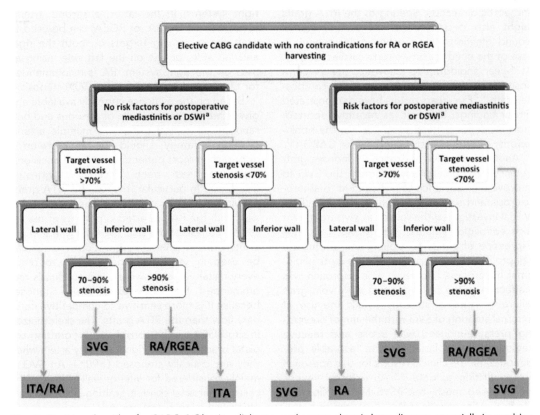

Fig. 2. Decision algorithm for CABG. [a] Obesity, diabetes, and severe chronic lung disease, especially in combination, are important clinical variables in the decision-making process. DSWI, deep sternal wound infection.

functional and an anatomic assessment of bypass grafts and to obtain a direct image of the flow through the coronary anastomosis.[157] In observational studies, the use of intraoperative graft assessment has been shown to reduce the rate of adverse events and graft failure, although interpretation can be challenging in sequential and T-graft configurations.[158–160]

Aortic manipulation

Atheroembolism is a major weakness of CABG vis-à-vis PCI. In a recent patient-level pooled analysis involving 11,518 patients, PCI was associated with reduced rates of periprocedural stroke; however, PCI and CABG were associated with a similar risk of stroke between 31 days and 5 years. The greater risk of stroke after CABG compared with PCI was confined to patients with MVD and diabetes.[161] Avoidance of aortic manipulation has been recommended by the recent guidelines to reduce the risk atheroembolism. Off-pump CABG (OPCABG) surgery may potentially avoid aortic cross-clamping and therefore minimize this risk. Several meta-analyses and the largest OPCABG randomized clinical trial demonstrated a reduction of the incidence of short-term

stroke with OPCABG compared with traditional on-pump CABG.[162,163] Further pooled analysis of high-risk subgroups confirmed the reduction in stroke incidence and demonstrated a survival benefit at the cost of increased need for repeated revascularization.[164] In clinical practice at many centers, however, side clamping of aorta to perform proximal anastomoses is still performed during OPCABG, which still exposes the patient to the risk of neurologic events caused by dislocation of hard or soft plaques.

These observations lead to 3 considerations. First, minimization of aortic manipulation is crucial to avoid cerebrovascular events. A propensity-matched analysis reported not only a lower rate of stroke but also a trend toward reduced in-hospital mortality when aortic clamping is avoided,[165] and, even in on-pump surgery, avoidance of multiple clamping or side-biting clamp techniques can help significantly.[2] Second, the use of devices allowing for clampless proximal anastomosis, especially in OPCABG, should be encouraged.[165–167] Third, use of full aortic no-touch technique is expected to further maximize outcomes in terms of major cerebrovascular events.[168] In this context, a very recent meta-

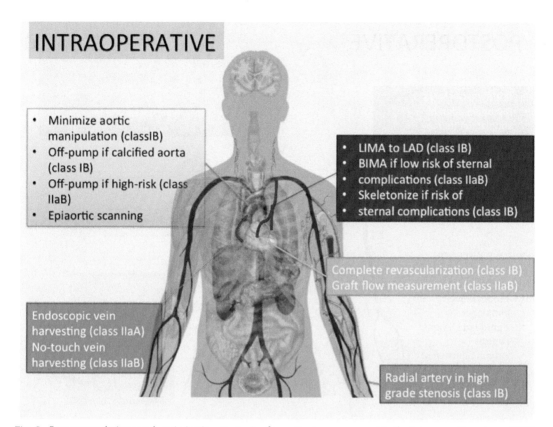

Fig. 3. Recommendations and optimization strategies for patient management in the intraoperative phase. BIMA, bilateral internal mammary artery; LIMA, left internal mammary artery.

analysis that included 13 studies and 37,720 subjects showed significant reductions in mortality, stroke, and renal failure when a no-touch, total arterial OPCABG technique was used.[169] Therefore, the weight of evidence supports the use of an anaortic technique using off-pump revascularization with only in situ ITA and composite (Y or T) grafts. Considering that intraoperative stroke has traditionally been the Achilles' heel of CABG in comparison with PCI, a broader use of the no-touch technique should be advocated in the surgical armamentarium.[11] This new direction of travel in CABG is supported by the finding of a similar incidence of stroke among the CABG and PCI arms of the EXCEL trial, in which surgeons were encouraged to use intraoperative ultrasound to guide cannulation and aortic manipulation.[170,171] The main limitation to the widespread application of the no-touch technique is its higher technical complexity.[68,172]

Minimally invasive surgery

Avoidance of median sternotomy by means of a small (5–10 cm) left anterior thoracotomy with rib-spreading to perform CABG, minimally invasive direct coronary artery bypass (MIDCAB),

has been proposed as an attractive alternative to standard CABG.[173] The LITA grafts can be harvested under direct vision or in video-assisted or robotic-assisted fashion, and CABG can be performed with intraoperative mortality of 0.8%, a 95.5% early graft patency rate, and 5-year and 10-year survival of 88.3% and 76.6%, respectively.[174] Another propensity-matched study confirmed rates of procedural complications and lengths of hospital stay after LAD revascularization via MIDCAB that were similar to those after sternotomy.[175] Overall, a safety and efficacy profile similar to conventional on-pump CABG and OPCABG intervention has been described in the literature, with an early quality of life benefit despite an increase in postoperative pain.[176–178] MIDCAB was shown to be particularly safe and effective for proximal LAD disease or a chronically occluded LAD.[179] When compared with PCI in the setting of single-vessel LAD disease, it was associated with a reduced need for repeated intervention.[180–182]

Based on these observations, a further evolution in surgical revascularization relies on the combination of MIDCAB LITA grafts to the LAD with PCI to the other vessels; that is, hybrid

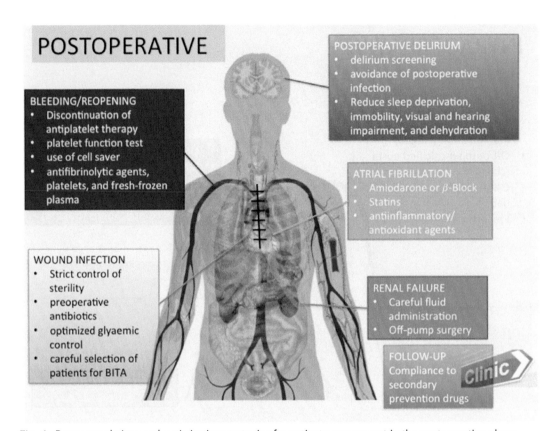

POSTOPERATIVE

BLEEDING/REOPENING
• Discontinuation of antiplatelet therapy
• platelet function test
• use of cell saver
• antifibrinolytic agents, platelets, and fresh-frozen plasma

POSTOPERATIVE DELIRIUM
• delirium screening
• avoidance of postoperative infection
• Reduce sleep deprivation, immobility, visual and hearing impairment, and dehydration

ATRIAL FIBRILLATION
• Amiodarone or β-Block
• Statins
• antiinflammatory/ antioxidant agents

WOUND INFECTION
• Strict control of sterility
• preoperative antibiotics
• optimized glyaemic control
• careful selection of patients for BITA

RENAL FAILURE
• Careful fluid administration
• Off-pump surgery

FOLLOW-UP
Compliance to secondary prevention drugs

Clinic

Fig. 4. Recommendations and optimization strategies for patient management in the postoperative phase.

coronary revascularization (HCR).[183] The 2 procedures can be performed at the same time in a hybrid operating room or in a sequential fashion.[184–186] A randomized trial that included 200 subjects showed no difference in terms of 1-year and 5-year rates of survival, MI, stroke, and major bleeding or repeat revascularization when compared with standard CABG.[187] Further benefits include a shorter recovery time and return-to-work time for the patients and higher satisfaction related to the avoidance of a sternotomy wound. However, despite the promising results, obstacles to the widespread application of this approach include concerns regarding patency rates, especially of non-LAD vessels,[188] and the relative paucity of candidates for this approach (only 0.5% of the patients between 2011 and 2013 in a large US database underwent HCR).[189] Criteria for HCR include a proximal LAD lesion that is graftable via a MIDCAB or a robotic MIDCAB procedure and a complexity of the remaining lesions amenable for PCI; that is, a low to intermediate SYNTAX score in the absence of contraindications for dual antiplatelet therapy. In attendance of more solid evidence on HRC over standard total arterial CABG, the indications for hybrid procedures remain restricted to patients with low SYNTAX score but an LAD lesion not amenable to PCI; patients with graftable proximal LAD lesion but poor surgical targets in the circumflex or right coronary artery but amenable to PCI; and patients with contraindications to sternotomy.

A large variation in the clinical practice of HCR has been reported, with approximately 12% of patients considered eligible for HCR in the recent Hybrid Coronary Observational Trial (NCT03089398) funded by the National Institutes of Health.[190] The Hybrid Coronary Revascularization Trial is a prospective, randomized trial of HCR versus multivessel PCI sponsored by the National Heart, Lung, and Blood Institute, which started enrollment in late 2017. This trial will randomize approximately 2350 subjects with low SYNTAX-scores to either sternal-sparing, off-pump, isolated LITA grafts to LAD revascularization combined with PCI to at least 1 non–left anterior descending target, or to multivessel PCI with drug-eluting stent, including the left anterior descending or left main coronary artery. The primary outcome is the composite of all-cause mortality, MI, stroke, or unplanned revascularization at 5-year follow-up.

Finally, totally endoscopic CABG is still limited by major technical issues with rate of conversions as high as 20%, emphasizing the need for newer more maneuverable anastomotic devices to improve outcomes.[191] **Fig. 3** summarizes the current recommendations in the intraoperative management of CAD patients and the proposed strategies to optimize their outcomes.

Postoperative Management

Postoperative complications mainly include reoperation for bleeding, renal failure, atrial fibrillation, delirium, mediastinitis, or wound infection. The incidence of reoperation for bleeding is around 2% to 4%; major risk factors include preoperative continuation of antiplatelet or anticoagulation therapy, urgency of the procedure, prior cardiovascular surgery, and the number of distal anastomoses. Useful measures to mitigate the reexploration risk are discontinuation of antiplatelet therapy or delaying surgery until optimization of platelet function is achieved. Also, use of cell saver, antifibrinolytic agents, platelets, and fresh-frozen plasma can reduce the need for reoperation.

A variable degree of kidney impairment is very common after CABG; however, dialysis is required in only in 1% of these cases. Risk factors include poor preoperative renal function, diabetes mellitus, and preoperative critical status.[2] As previously discussed, it seems that OPCABG surgery is effective in reducing the risk of renal failure; however, careful management of fluid administration in intensive care environments is also advocated.

Atrial fibrillation is a common arrhythmia postoperatively (occurring in approximatively 15%–30% of cases) that is easily treatable with amiodarone or sotalol. However, antiinflammatory corticosteroids; β-blockers statins; and antioxidant agents, such as N-acetylcysteine, ACE inhibitors, and omega-3 fatty acids, might have a protective role. Peripheral vascular disease, preoperative atrial fibrillation, and obesity are considered predictors of its occurrence.

Delirium is normally associated with older age, previous poor cognitive function, or cerebrovascular disease and duration of cardiopulmonary bypass. Preoperative delirium screening, avoidance of postoperative infection, and a multilevel intervention to reduce sleep deprivation, immobility, visual and hearing impairment, and dehydration are thought to attenuate the rate of its occurrence.

Wound infection and mediastinitis have an incidence of 0.5% to 2%. Obesity, diabetes mellitus, hypertension, and preoperative renal failure on dialysis are clinical variables predicting its occurrence. Also, redo surgery, duration of cardiopulmonary bypass, use of nonskeletonized BITA, or postoperative reexploration for bleeding represent significant risks factors for this complication. Strict control of sterility, preoperative antibiotics, optimized glycemic control, and careful selection of patients for BITA are important in mitigating the risk of mediastinitis.

Strict compliance to antiplatelet medications, β-blockers, statins, and angiotensin-converting enzyme inhibitors after CABG should be encouraged to significantly improve long-term outcomes as shown in a recent meta-analysis investigating the current compliance with guideline-directed medical therapy in coronary revascularization trials.[192] **Fig. 4** summarizes the currently suggested interventions to minimize postoperative complications risk.

SUMMARY

CABG represents the mainstay in the treatment of multivessel coronary disease and, despite the increasing risk profile of the referred patients, this procedure can be performed safely with low rates of complications and good long-term outcomes. Multiple arterial grafting, especially if associated with anaortic techniques, might provide the best longer-term outcomes. Individualization to the patients' clinical characteristics and the experience of the surgeon and the team are key to excellent outcomes.

REFERENCES

1. Bang VV, Levy MS. In multivessel coronary artery disease, a "state-of-the-art" randomized clinical trial of revascularization is needed. Catheter Cardiovasc Interv 2016;87(1):13–4.
2. Head SJ, Milojevic M, Taggart DP, et al. Current practice of state-of-the-art surgical coronary revascularization. Circulation 2017;136(14):1331–45.
3. Mohr FW, Morice MC, Kappetein AP, et al. Coronary artery bypass graft surgery versus percutaneous coronary intervention in patients with three-vessel disease and left main coronary disease: 5-year follow-up of the randomised, clinical SYNTAX trial. Lancet 2013;381(9867):629–38.
4. Sousa-Uva M, Neumann FJ, Ahlsson A, et al. 2018 ESC/EACTS guidelines on myocardial revascularization. Eur J Cardiothorac Surg 2018. https://doi.org/10.1093/ejcts/ezy289.
5. ElBardissi AW, Aranki SF, Sheng S, et al. Trends in isolated coronary artery bypass grafting: an analysis of the Society of Thoracic Surgeons adult cardiac surgery database. J Thorac Cardiovasc Surg 2012;143(2):273–81.

6. Edwards FH, Ferraris VA, Kurlansky PA, et al. Failure to rescue rates after coronary artery bypass grafting: an analysis from the Society of Thoracic Surgeons adult cardiac surgery database. Ann Thorac Surg 2016;102(2):458–64.

7. Taggart DP, Altman DG, Gray AM, et al. Randomized trial to compare bilateral vs. single internal mammary coronary artery bypass grafting: 1-year results of the Arterial Revascularisation Trial (ART). Eur Heart J 2010;31(20):2470–81.

8. Lamy A, Devereaux PJ, Prabhakaran D, et al. Off-pump or on-pump coronary-artery bypass grafting at 30 days. N Engl J Med 2012;366(16):1489–97.

9. Head SJ, Milojevic M, Daemen J, et al. Mortality after coronary artery bypass grafting versus percutaneous coronary intervention with stenting for coronary artery disease: a pooled analysis of individual patient data. Lancet 2018;391(10124): 939–48.

10. Spadaccio C, Benedetto U. Coronary artery bypass grafting (CABG) vs. percutaneous coronary intervention (PCI) in the treatment of multivessel coronary disease: quo vadis? -a review of the evidences on coronary artery disease. Ann Cardiothorac Surg 2018;7(4):506–15.

11. Gaudino M, Taggart DP. What is new in the armamentarium of coronary surgeons to compete with PCI? EuroIntervention 2018;14(4):e387–9.

12. Nashef SA, Roques F, Sharples LD, et al. EuroSCORE II. Eur J Cardiothorac Surg 2012;41(4): 734–44 [discussion: 744–5].

13. Shahian DM, O'Brien SM, Filardo G, et al. The Society of Thoracic Surgeons 2008 cardiac surgery risk models: part 3–valve plus coronary artery bypass grafting surgery. Ann Thorac Surg 2009; 88(1 Suppl):S43–62.

14. Wang TK, Li AY, Ramanathan T, et al. Comparison of four risk scores for contemporary isolated coronary artery bypass grafting. Heart Lung Circ 2014; 23(5):469–74.

15. Kappetein AP, Head SJ, Genereux P, et al. Updated standardized endpoint definitions for transcatheter aortic valve implantation: the Valve Academic Research Consortium-2 consensus document. J Thorac Cardiovasc Surg 2013; 145(1):6–23.

16. Kolh P, Windecker S, Alfonso F, et al. 2014 ESC/EACTS guidelines on myocardial revascularization: the task force on myocardial revascularization of the European Society of Cardiology (ESC) and the European Association for Cardio-Thoracic Surgery (EACTS). Developed with the special contribution of the European Association of Percutaneous Cardiovascular Interventions (EAPCI). Eur J Cardiothorac Surg 2014;46(4):517–92.

17. Hillis LD, Smith PK, Anderson JL, et al. 2011 ACCF/AHA guideline for coronary artery bypass graft surgery: a report of the American College of Cardiology Foundation/American Heart Association Task Force on practice guidelines. Circulation 2011;124(23):e652–735.

18. De Bruyne B, Pijls NH, Kalesan B, et al. Fractional flow reserve-guided PCI versus medical therapy in stable coronary disease. N Engl J Med 2012; 367(11):991–1001.

19. Fearon WF, Nishi T, De Bruyne B, et al. Clinical outcomes and cost-effectiveness of fractional flow reserve-guided percutaneous coronary intervention in patients with stable coronary artery disease: three-year follow-up of the FAME 2 trial (fractional flow reserve versus angiography for multivessel evaluation). Circulation 2018;137(5): 480–7.

20. Adjedj J, De Bruyne B, Flore V, et al. Significance of intermediate values of fractional flow reserve in patients with coronary artery disease. Circulation 2016;133(5):502–8.

21. De Bruyne B, Fearon WF, Pijls NH, et al. Fractional flow reserve-guided PCI for stable coronary artery disease. N Engl J Med 2014;371(13):1208–17.

22. Tonino PA, Fearon WF, De Bruyne B, et al. Angiographic versus functional severity of coronary artery stenoses in the FAME study fractional flow reserve versus angiography in multivessel evaluation. J Am Coll Cardiol 2010;55(25):2816–21.

23. Botman CJ, Schonberger J, Koolen S, et al. Does stenosis severity of native vessels influence bypass graft patency? A prospective fractional flow reserve-guided study. Ann Thorac Surg 2007; 83(6):2093–7.

24. Cosgrove DM, Loop FD, Saunders CL, et al. Should coronary arteries with less than fifty percent stenosis be bypassed? J Thorac Cardiovasc Surg 1981;82(4):520–30.

25. Toth G, De Bruyne B, Casselman F, et al. Fractional flow reserve-guided versus angiography-guided coronary artery bypass graft surgery. Circulation 2013;128(13):1405–11.

26. Shaw LJ, Berman DS, Maron DJ, et al. Optimal medical therapy with or without percutaneous coronary intervention to reduce ischemic burden: results from the Clinical Outcomes Utilizing Revascularization and Aggressive Drug Evaluation (COURAGE) trial nuclear substudy. Circulation 2008;117(10):1283–91.

27. Garcia S, Sandoval Y, Roukoz H, et al. Outcomes after complete versus incomplete revascularization of patients with multivessel coronary artery disease: a meta-analysis of 89,883 patients enrolled in randomized clinical trials and observational studies. J Am Coll Cardiol 2013;62(16):1421–31.

28. Farooq V, Serruys PW, Garcia-Garcia HM, et al. The negative impact of incomplete angiographic revascularization on clinical outcomes and its

association with total occlusions: the SYNTAX (Synergy Between Percutaneous Coronary Intervention with Taxus and Cardiac Surgery) trial. J Am Coll Cardiol 2013;61(3):282–94.

29. Ahn JM, Park DW, Lee CW, et al. Comparison of stenting versus bypass surgery according to the completeness of revascularization in severe coronary artery disease: patient-level pooled analysis of the SYNTAX, PRECOMBAT, and BEST trials. JACC Cardiovasc Interv 2017;10(14):1415–24.

30. Milojevic M, Head SJ, Parasca CA, et al. Causes of death following PCI versus CABG in complex CAD: 5-year follow-up of SYNTAX. J Am Coll Cardiol 2016;67(1):42–55.

31. Nappi F, Sutherland FW, Al-Attar N, et al. Incomplete revascularization in PCI and CABG: when two plus two does not make four. J Am Coll Cardiol 2016;68(8):877–8.

32. Benedetto U, Gaudino M, Di Franco A, et al. Incomplete revascularization and long-term survival after coronary artery bypass surgery. Int J Cardiol 2018;254:59–63.

33. Head SJ, Davierwala PM, Serruys PW, et al. Coronary artery bypass grafting vs. percutaneous coronary intervention for patients with three-vessel disease: final five-year follow-up of the SYNTAX trial. Eur Heart J 2014;35(40):2821–30.

34. Morice MC, Serruys PW, Kappetein AP, et al. Five-year outcomes in patients with left main disease treated with either percutaneous coronary intervention or coronary artery bypass grafting in the synergy between percutaneous coronary intervention with taxus and cardiac surgery trial. Circulation 2014;129(23):2388–94.

35. Cavalcante R, Sotomi Y, Zeng Y, et al. Coronary bypass surgery versus stenting in multivessel disease involving the proximal left anterior descending coronary artery. Heart 2017;103(6):428–33.

36. Chang M, Ahn JM, Lee CW, et al. Long-term mortality after coronary revascularization in nondiabetic patients with multivessel disease. J Am Coll Cardiol 2016;68(1):29–36.

37. Velazquez EJ, Lee KL, Jones RH, et al. Coronary-artery bypass surgery in patients with ischemic cardiomyopathy. N Engl J Med 2016;374(16):1511–20.

38. Petrie MC, Jhund PS, She L, et al. Ten-year outcomes after coronary artery bypass grafting according to age in patients with heart failure and left ventricular systolic dysfunction: an analysis of the extended follow-up of the STICH trial (Surgical Treatment for Ischemic Heart Failure). Circulation 2016;134(18):1314–24.

39. Stone GW, Sabik JF, Serruys PW, et al. Everolimus-eluting stents or bypass surgery for left main coronary artery disease. N Engl J Med 2016;375(23):2223–35.

40. Makikallio T, Holm NR, Lindsay M, et al. Percutaneous coronary angioplasty versus coronary artery bypass grafting in treatment of unprotected left main stenosis (NOBLE): a prospective, randomised, open-label, non-inferiority trial. Lancet 2016;388(10061):2743–52.

41. Giacoppo D, Colleran R, Cassese S, et al. Percutaneous coronary intervention vs coronary artery bypass grafting in patients with left main coronary artery stenosis: a systematic review and meta-analysis. JAMA Cardiol 2017;2(10):1079–88.

42. Freemantle N, Ruel M, Gaudino MFL, et al. On the pooling and subgrouping of data from percutaneous coronary intervention versus coronary artery bypass grafting trials: a call to circumspection. Eur J Cardiothorac Surg 2018;53(5):915–8.

43. Loop FD, Lytle BW, Cosgrove DM, et al. Influence of the internal-mammary-artery graft on 10-year survival and other cardiac events. N Engl J Med 1986;314(1):1–6.

44. Boylan MJ, Lytle BW, Loop FD, et al. Surgical treatment of isolated left anterior descending coronary stenosis. Comparison of left internal mammary artery and venous autograft at 18 to 20 years of follow-up. J Thorac Cardiovasc Surg 1994;107(3):657–62.

45. Otsuka F, Yahagi K, Sakakura K, et al. Why is the mammary artery so special and what protects it from atherosclerosis? Ann Cardiothorac Surg 2013;2(4):519–26.

46. Gaudino M, Antoniades C, Benedetto U, et al. Mechanisms, consequences, and prevention of coronary graft failure. Circulation 2017;136(18):1749–64.

47. Henriquez-Pino JA, Gomes WJ, Prates JC, et al. Surgical anatomy of the internal thoracic artery. Ann Thorac Surg 1997;64(4):1041–5.

48. Dai C, Lu Z, Zhu H, et al. Bilateral internal mammary artery grafting and risk of sternal wound infection: evidence from observational studies. Ann Thorac Surg 2013;95(6):1938–45.

49. Deo SV, Shah IK, Dunlay SM, et al. Bilateral internal thoracic artery harvest and deep sternal wound infection in diabetic patients. Ann Thorac Surg 2013;95(3):862–9.

50. Sa MP, Ferraz PE, Escobar RR, et al. Skeletonized versus pedicled internal thoracic artery and risk of sternal wound infection after coronary bypass surgery: meta-analysis and meta-regression of 4817 patients. Interact Cardiovasc Thorac Surg 2013;16(6):849–57.

51. Sa MP, Cavalcanti PE, Santos HJ, et al. Flow capacity of skeletonized versus pedicled internal thoracic artery in coronary artery bypass graft surgery: systematic review, meta-analysis and meta-regression. Eur J Cardiothorac Surg 2015;48(1):25–31.

52. Martinez-Gonzalez B, Reyes-Hernandez CG, Quir-oga-Garza A, et al. Conduits used in coronary artery bypass grafting: a review of morphological studies. Ann Thorac Cardiovasc Surg 2017;23(2):55–65.

53. Tatoulis J, Buxton BF, Fuller JA. The right internal thoracic artery: is it underutilized? Curr Opin Cardiol 2011;26(6):528–35.

54. Lopes RD, Mehta RH, Hafley GE, et al. Relationship between vein graft failure and subsequent clinical outcomes after coronary artery bypass surgery. Circulation 2012;125(6):749–56.

55. Baikoussis NG, Papakonstantinou NA, Apostolakis E. Radial artery as graft for coronary artery bypass surgery: advantages and disadvantages for its usage focused on structural and biological characteristics. J Cardiol 2014;63(5):321–8.

56. Yi G, Shine B, Rehman SM, et al. Effect of bilateral internal mammary artery grafts on long-term survival: a meta-analysis approach. Circulation 2014; 130(7):539–45.

57. Schwann TA, Habib RH, Wallace A, et al. Operative outcomes of multiple-arterial versus single-arterial coronary bypass grafting. Ann Thorac Surg 2018;105(4):1109–19.

58. Taggart DP, D'Amico R, Altman DG. Effect of arterial revascularisation on survival: a systematic review of studies comparing bilateral and single internal mammary arteries. Lancet 2001; 358(9285):870–5.

59. Weiss AJ, Zhao S, Tian DH, et al. A meta-analysis comparing bilateral internal mammary artery with left internal mammary artery for coronary artery bypass grafting. Ann Cardiothorac Surg 2013; 2(4):390–400.

60. Kurlansky PA, Traad EA, Dorman MJ, et al. Thirty-year follow-up defines survival benefit for second internal mammary artery in propensity-matched groups. Ann Thorac Surg 2010;90(1):101–8.

61. Dorman MJ, Kurlansky PA, Traad EA, et al. Bilateral internal mammary artery grafting enhances survival in diabetic patients: a 30-year follow-up of propensity score-matched cohorts. Circulation 2012;126(25):2935–42.

62. Galbut DL, Kurlansky PA, Traad EA, et al. Bilateral internal thoracic artery grafting improves long-term survival in patients with reduced ejection fraction: a propensity-matched study with 30-year follow-up. J Thorac Cardiovasc Surg 2012; 143(4):844–53.e4.

63. Grau JB, Ferrari G, Mak AW, et al. Propensity matched analysis of bilateral internal mammary artery versus single left internal mammary artery grafting at 17-year follow-up: validation of a contemporary surgical experience. Eur J Cardiothorac Surg 2012;41(4):770–5 [discussion: 776].

64. Lytle BW. Bilateral internal thoracic artery grafting. Ann Cardiothorac Surg 2013;2(4):485–92.

65. Rubino AS, Gatti G, Reichart D, et al. Early outcome of bilateral versus single internal mammary artery grafting in the elderly. Ann Thorac Surg 2018;105(6):1717–23.

66. Kieser TM, Lewin AM, Graham MM, et al. Outcomes associated with bilateral internal thoracic artery grafting: the importance of age. Ann Thorac Surg 2011;92(4):1269–75 [discussion: 1275–6].

67. Mohammadi S, Dagenais F, Doyle D, et al. Age cut-off for the loss of benefit from bilateral internal thoracic artery grafting. Eur J Cardiothorac Surg 2008;33(6):977–82.

68. Gaudino M, Bakaeen F, Benedetto U, et al. Use rate and outcome in bilateral internal thoracic artery grafting: insights from a systematic review and meta-analysis. J Am Heart Assoc 2018;7(11) [pii:e009361].

69. Taggart DP, Altman DG, Gray AM, et al. Randomized trial of bilateral versus single internal-thoracic-artery grafts. N Engl J Med 2016; 375(26):2540–9.

70. Benedetto U, Altman DG, Gerry S, et al. Pedicled and skeletonized single and bilateral internal thoracic artery grafts and the incidence of sternal wound complications: insights from the arterial revascularization trial. J Thorac Cardiovasc Surg 2016;152(1):270–6.

71. Royse A, Eccleston D, Royse C, et al. Bilateral versus single internal-thoracic-artery grafts. N Engl J Med 2017;376(18):e37.

72. Gaudino M, Tranbaugh R, Fremes S. Bilateral versus single internal-thoracic-artery grafts. N Engl J Med 2017;376(18):e37.

73. Raza S, Blackstone EH, Sabik JF III. Bilateral versus single internal-thoracic-artery grafts. N Engl J Med 2017;376(18):e37.

74. Gaudino M, Di Franco A, Rahouma M, et al. Unmeasured confounders in observational studies comparing bilateral versus single internal thoracic artery for coronary artery bypass grafting: a meta-analysis. J Am Heart Assoc 2018;7(1) [pii:e008010].

75. Gaudino MFL, Taggart DP, Fremes SE. The ROMA trial: why it is needed. Curr Opin Cardiol 2018;33(6):622–6.

76. Carpentier A, Guermonprez JL, Deloche A, et al. The aorta-to-coronary radial artery bypass graft. A technique avoiding pathological changes in grafts. Ann Thorac Surg 1973;16(2):111–21.

77. Myers MG, Fremes SE. Prevention of radial artery graft spasm: a survey of Canadian surgical centres. Can J Cardiol 2003;19(6):677–81.

78. Gaudino M, Prati F, Caradonna E, et al. Implantation in coronary circulation induces morphofunctional transformation of radial grafts from muscular to elastomuscular. Circulation 2005; 112(9 Suppl):I208–11.

79. Patel A, Asopa S, Dunning J. Should patients receiving a radial artery conduit have post-operative calcium channel blockers? Interact Cardiovasc Thorac Surg 2006;5(3):251–7.

80. Acar C, Jebara VA, Portoghese M, et al. Revival of the radial artery for coronary artery bypass grafting. Ann Thorac Surg 1992;54(4):652–9 [discussion: 659–60].

81. Tatoulis J, Buxton BF, Fuller JA, et al. Long-term patency of 1108 radial arterial-coronary angiograms over 10 years. Ann Thorac Surg 2009; 88(1):23–9 [discussion 29–30].

82. Gaudino M, Tondi P, Benedetto U, et al. Radial artery as a coronary artery bypass conduit: 20-year results. J Am Coll Cardiol 2016;68(6):603–10.

83. Gaudino M, Benedetto U, Fremes S, et al. Radial-artery or saphenous-vein grafts in coronary-artery bypass surgery. N Engl J Med 2018;378(22): 2069–77.

84. Deb S, Cohen EA, Singh SK, et al. Radial artery and saphenous vein patency more than 5 years after coronary artery bypass surgery: results from RAPS (Radial Artery Patency Study). J Am Coll Cardiol 2012;60(1):28–35.

85. Goldman S, Sethi GK, Holman W, et al. Radial artery grafts vs saphenous vein grafts in coronary artery bypass surgery: a randomized trial. JAMA 2011;305(2):167–74.

86. Collins P, Webb CM, Chong CF, et al. Radial artery versus saphenous vein patency trial i. radial artery versus saphenous vein patency randomized trial: five-year angiographic follow-up. Circulation 2008;117(22):2859–64.

87. Hayward PA, Buxton BF. Mid-term results of the radial artery patency and clinical outcomes randomized trial. Ann Cardiothorac Surg 2013;2(4): 458–66.

88. Benedetto U, Angeloni E, Refice S, et al. Radial artery versus saphenous vein graft patency: meta-analysis of randomized controlled trials. J Thorac Cardiovasc Surg 2010;139(1):229–31.

89. Athanasiou T, Saso S, Rao C, et al. Radial artery versus saphenous vein conduits for coronary artery bypass surgery: forty years of competition– which conduit offers better patency? A systematic review and meta-analysis. Eur J Cardiothorac Surg 2011;40(1):208–20.

90. Cao C, Manganas C, Horton M, et al. Angiographic outcomes of radial artery versus saphenous vein in coronary artery bypass graft surgery: a meta-analysis of randomized controlled trials. J Thorac Cardiovasc Surg 2013;146(2): 255–61.

91. Zhang H, Wang ZW, Wu HB, et al. Radial artery graft vs. saphenous vein graft for coronary artery bypass surgery: which conduit offers better efficacy? Herz 2014;39(4):458–65.

92. Benedetto U, Raja SG, Albanese A, et al. Searching for the second best graft for coronary artery bypass surgery: a network meta-analysis of randomized controlled trialsdagger. Eur J Cardiothorac Surg 2015;47(1):59–65 [discussion: 65].

93. Benedetto U, Gaudino M, Caputo M, et al. Right internal thoracic artery versus radial artery as the second best arterial conduit: insights from a meta-analysis of propensity-matched data on long-term survival. J Thorac Cardiovasc Surg 2016;152(4):1083–91.e15.

94. Hu X, Zhao Q. Systematic comparison of the effectiveness of radial artery and saphenous vein or right internal thoracic artery coronary bypass grafts in non-left anterior descending coronary arteries. J Zhejiang Univ Sci B 2011;12(4):273–9.

95. Hoffman DM, Dimitrova KR, Lucido DJ, et al. Optimal conduit for diabetic patients: propensity analysis of radial and right internal thoracic arteries. Ann Thorac Surg 2014;98(1):30–6 [discussion: 36–7].

96. Tranbaugh RF, Dimitrova KR, Lucido DJ, et al. The second best arterial graft: a propensity analysis of the radial artery versus the free right internal thoracic artery to bypass the circumflex coronary artery. J Thorac Cardiovasc Surg 2014;147(1):133–40.

97. Amano A, Takahashi A, Hirose H. Skeletonized radial artery grafting: improved angiographic results. Ann Thorac Surg 2002;73(6):1880–7.

98. Rukosujew A, Reichelt R, Fabricius AM, et al. Skeletonization versus pedicle preparation of the radial artery with and without the ultrasonic scalpel. Ann Thorac Surg 2004;77(1):120–5.

99. Gaudino M, Crea F, Cammertoni F, et al. Technical issues in the use of the radial artery as a coronary artery bypass conduit. Ann Thorac Surg 2014;98(6):2247–54.

100. Navia JL, Olivares G, Ehasz P, et al. Endoscopic radial artery harvesting procedure for coronary artery bypass grafting. Ann Cardiothorac Surg 2013; 2(4):557–64.

101. Cao C, Tian DH, Ang SC, et al. A meta-analysis of endoscopic versus conventional open radial artery harvesting for coronary artery bypass graft surgery. Innovations (Phila) 2014;9(4):269–75.

102. Gaudino M, Alessandrini F, Pragliola C, et al. Effect of target artery location and severity of stenosis on mid-term patency of aorta-anastomosed vs. internal thoracic artery-anastomosed radial artery grafts. Eur J Cardiothorac Surg 2004;25(3):424–8.

103. Benedetto U, Caputo M, Zakkar M, et al. Are three arteries better than two? Impact of using the radial artery in addition to bilateral internal thoracic artery grafting on long-term survival. J Thorac Cardiovasc Surg 2016;152(3):862–9. e2.

104. Grau JB, Kuschner CE, Johnson CK, et al. The effects of using a radial artery in patients already

receiving bilateral internal mammary arteries during coronary bypass grafting: 30-day outcomes and 14-year survival in a propensity-matched cohort. Eur J Cardiothorac Surg 2016;49(1): 203–10.

105. Shi WY, Tatoulis J, Newcomb AE, et al. Is a third arterial conduit necessary? Comparison of the radial artery and saphenous vein in patients receiving bilateral internal thoracic arteries for triple vessel coronary disease. Eur J Cardiothorac Surg 2016;50(1):53–60.

106. Gaudino M, Puskas JD, Di Franco A, et al. Three arterial grafts improve late survival: a meta-analysis of propensity-matched studies. Circulation 2017;135(11):1036–44.

107. Yanagawa B, Verma S, Mazine A, et al. Impact of total arterial revascularization on long term survival: a systematic review and meta-analysis of 130,305 patients. Int J Cardiol 2017;233:29–36.

108. Jarvis MA, Jarvis CL, Jones PR, et al. Reliability of Allen's test in selection of patients for radial artery harvest. Ann Thorac Surg 2000;70(4):1362–5.

109. Gaudino M, Leone A, Lupascu A, et al. Morphological and functional consequences of transradial coronary angiography on the radial artery: implications for its use as a bypass conduit. Eur J Cardiothorac Surg 2015;48(3):370–4.

110. Gaudino M, Burzotta F, Bakaeen F, et al. The radial artery for percutaneous coronary procedures or surgery? J Am Coll Cardiol 2018;71(10): 1167–75.

111. van Son JA, Smedts F, Vincent JG, et al. Comparative anatomic studies of various arterial conduits for myocardial revascularization. J Thorac Cardiovasc Surg 1990;99(4):703–7.

112. Suma H. The right gastroepiploic artery graft for coronary artery bypass grafting: a 30-year experience. Korean J Thorac Cardiovasc Surg 2016; 49(4):225–31.

113. Pym J, Brown PM, Charrette EJ, et al. Gastroepiploic-coronary anastomosis. A viable alternative bypass graft. J Thorac Cardiovasc Surg 1987; 94(2):256–9.

114. Suma H, Fukumoto H, Takeuchi A. Coronary artery bypass grafting by utilizing in situ right gastroepiploic artery: basic study and clinical application. Ann Thorac Surg 1987;44(4):394–7.

115. Takayama T, Suma H, Wanibuchi Y, et al. Physiological and pharmacological responses of arterial graft flow after coronary artery bypass grafting measured with an implantable ultrasonic Doppler miniprobe. Circulation 1992;86(5 Suppl):II217–23.

116. Ochiai M, Ohno M, Taguchi J, et al. Responses of human gastroepiploic arteries to vasoactive substances: comparison with responses of internal mammary arteries and saphenous veins. J Thorac Cardiovasc Surg 1992;104(2):453–8.

117. Suma H, Takanashi R. Arteriosclerosis of the gastroepiploic and internal thoracic arteries. Ann Thorac Surg 1990;50(3):413–6.

118. Saito T, Suma H, Terada Y, et al. Availability of the in situ right gastroepiploic artery for coronary artery bypass. Ann Thorac Surg 1992;53(2):266–8.

119. Suma H, Wanibuchi Y, Furuta S, et al. Does use of gastroepiploic artery graft increase surgical risk? J Thorac Cardiovasc Surg 1991;101(1):121–5.

120. Hillis LD, Smith PK, Anderson JL, et al. 2011 ACCF/AHA guideline for coronary artery bypass graft surgery. a report of the American College of Cardiology Foundation/American Heart Association Task Force on practice guidelines. Developed in collaboration with the American Association for Thoracic Surgery, Society of Cardiovascular Anesthesiologists, and Society of Thoracic Surgeons. J Am Coll Cardiol 2011; 58(24):e123–210.

121. Suzuki T, Asai T, Nota H, et al. Early and long-term patency of in situ skeletonized gastroepiploic artery after off-pump coronary artery bypass graft surgery. Ann Thorac Surg 2013;96(1):90–5.

122. Suma H, Tanabe H, Takahashi A, et al. Twenty years experience with the gastroepiploic artery graft for CABG. Circulation 2007;116(11 Suppl):I188–91.

123. Glineur D, D'Hoore W, Price J, et al. Survival benefit of multiple arterial grafting in a 25-year single-institutional experience: the importance of the third arterial graft. Eur J Cardiothorac Surg 2012;42(2):284–90 [discussion: 290–1].

124. Suzuki T, Asai T, Matsubayashi K, et al. In off-pump surgery, skeletonized gastroepiploic artery is superior to saphenous vein in patients with bilateral internal thoracic arterial grafts. Ann Thorac Surg 2011;91(4):1159–64.

125. Pevni D, Uretzky G, Yosef P, et al. Revascularization of the right coronary artery in bilateral internal thoracic artery grafting. Ann Thorac Surg 2005; 79(2):564–9.

126. Hwang HY, Cho KR, Kim KB. Equivalency of right internal thoracic artery and right gastroepiploic artery composite grafts: five-year outcomes. Ann Thorac Surg 2013;96(6):2061–8.

127. Motwani JG, Topol EJ. Aortocoronary saphenous vein graft disease: pathogenesis, predisposition, and prevention. Circulation 1998;97(9):916–31.

128. Allaire E, Clowes AW. Endothelial cell injury in cardiovascular surgery: the intimal hyperplastic response. Ann Thorac Surg 1997;63(2):582–91.

129. Spadaccio C, Nappi F, Al-Attar N, et al. CURRENT DEVELOPMENTS IN DRUG ELUTING DEVICES: introductory editorial: drug-eluting stents or drug-eluting grafts? insights from proteomic analysis. Drug Target Insights 2016;10(Suppl 1):15–9.

130. Hess CN, Lopes RD, Gibson CM, et al. Saphenous vein graft failure after coronary artery bypass

surgery: insights from PREVENT IV. Circulation 2014;130(17):1445–51.

131. Souza D. A new no-touch preparation technique. Technical notes. Scand J Thorac Cardiovasc Surg 1996;30(1):41–4.

132. Verma S, Lovren F, Pan Y, et al. Pedicled no-touch saphenous vein graft harvest limits vascular smooth muscle cell activation: the PATENT saphenous vein graft study. Eur J Cardiothorac Surg 2014;45(4):717–25.

133. Dreifaldt M, Souza D, Bodin L, et al. The vasa vasorum and associated endothelial nitric oxide synthase is more important for saphenous vein than arterial bypass grafts. Angiology 2013;64(4):293–9.

134. Samano N, Geijer H, Liden M, et al. The no-touch saphenous vein for coronary artery bypass grafting maintains a patency, after 16 years, comparable to the left internal thoracic artery: a randomized trial. J Thorac Cardiovasc Surg 2015;150(4):880–8.

135. Kopjar T, Dashwood MR. Endoscopic versus "no-touch" saphenous vein harvesting for coronary artery bypass grafting: a trade-off between wound healing and graft patency. Angiology 2016;67(2):121–32.

136. van Diepen S, Brennan JM, Hafley GE, et al. Endoscopic harvesting device type and outcomes in patients undergoing coronary artery bypass surgery. Ann Surg 2014;260(2):402–8.

137. Sastry P, Rivinius R, Harvey R, et al. The influence of endoscopic vein harvesting on outcomes after coronary bypass grafting: a meta-analysis of 267,525 patients. Eur J Cardiothorac Surg 2013;44(6):980–9.

138. Lopes RD, Hafley GE, Allen KB, et al. Endoscopic versus open vein-graft harvesting in coronary-artery bypass surgery. N Engl J Med 2009;361(3):235–44.

139. Rousou LJ, Taylor KB, Lu XG, et al. Saphenous vein conduits harvested by endoscopic technique exhibit structural and functional damage. Ann Thorac Surg 2009;87(1):62–70.

140. Deppe AC, Liakopoulos OJ, Choi YH, et al. Endoscopic vein harvesting for coronary artery bypass grafting: a systematic review with meta-analysis of 27,789 patients. J Surg Res 2013;180(1):114–24.

141. Williams JB, Peterson ED, Brennan JM, et al. Association between endoscopic vs open vein-graft harvesting and mortality, wound complications, and cardiovascular events in patients undergoing CABG surgery. JAMA 2012;308(5):475–84.

142. Shroyer AL, Grover FL, Hattler B, et al. On-pump versus off-pump coronary-artery bypass surgery. N Engl J Med 2009;361(19):1827–37.

143. Zenati MA, Shroyer AL, Collins JF, et al. Impact of endoscopic versus open saphenous vein harvest technique on late coronary artery bypass grafting patient outcomes in the ROOBY (Randomized On/Off Bypass) trial. J Thorac Cardiovasc Surg 2011;141(2):338–44.

144. Kim KB, Hwang HY, Hahn S, et al. A randomized comparison of the Saphenous Vein Versus Right Internal Thoracic Artery as a Y-Composite Graft (SAVE RITA) trial: one-year angiographic results and mid-term clinical outcomes. J Thorac Cardiovasc Surg 2014;148(3):901–7 [discussion: 907–8].

145. Hwang HY, Kim JS, Oh SJ, et al. A randomized comparison of the Saphenous Vein Versus Right Internal Thoracic Artery as a Y-Composite Graft (SAVE RITA) trial: early results. J Thorac Cardiovasc Surg 2012;144(5):1027–33.

146. Tedoriya T, Kawasuji M, Sakakibara N, et al. Pressure characteristics in arterial grafts for coronary bypass surgery. Cardiovasc Surg 1995;3(4):381–5.

147. Gaudino M, Fremes SE. The SAVE RITA trial at 5 years: more evidence is needed to transform a vein to an artery. J Thorac Cardiovasc Surg 2018;156(4):1434–5.

148. Alexander JH, Hafley G, Harrington RA, et al. Efficacy and safety of edifoligide, an E2F transcription factor decoy, for prevention of vein graft failure following coronary artery bypass graft surgery: PREVENT IV: a randomized controlled trial. JAMA 2005;294(19):2446–54.

149. Mawhinney JA, Mounsey CA, Taggart DP. The potential role of external venous supports in coronary artery bypass graft surgery. Eur J Cardiothorac Surg 2018;53(6):1127–34.

150. Inderbitzin DT, Bremerich J, Matt P, et al. One-year patency control and risk analysis of eSVS(R)-mesh-supported coronary saphenous vein grafts. J Cardiothorac Surg 2015;10:108.

151. Taggart DP, Amin S, Djordjevic J, et al. A prospective study of external stenting of saphenous vein grafts to the right coronary artery: the VEST II study. Eur J Cardiothorac Surg 2017;51(5):952–8.

152. Amin S, Werner RS, Madsen PL, et al. Influence of external stenting on venous graft flow parameters in coronary artery bypass grafting: a randomized study. Interact Cardiovasc Thorac Surg 2018;26(6):926–31.

153. Gaudino M, Alexander JH, Bakaeen FG, et al. Randomized comparison of the clinical outcome of single versus multiple arterial grafts: the ROMA trial-rationale and study protocol. Eur J Cardiothorac Surg 2017;52(6):1031–40.

154. Gaudino M, Taggart D, Suma H, et al. The choice of conduits in coronary artery bypass surgery. J Am Coll Cardiol 2015;66(15):1729–37.

155. Mujanovic E, Kabil E, Bergsland J. Transit time flowmetry in coronary surgery–an important tool in graft verification. Bosn J Basic Med Sci 2007;7(3):275–8.

156. Kieser TM, Rose S, Kowalewski R, et al. Transit-time flow predicts outcomes in coronary artery bypass graft patients: a series of 1000 consecutive arterial grafts. Eur J Cardiothorac Surg 2010;38(2): 155–62.

157. Di Giammarco G, Canosa C, Foschi M, et al. Intra-operative graft verification in coronary surgery: increased diagnostic accuracy adding high-resolution epicardial ultrasonography to transit-time flow measurement. Eur J Cardiothorac Surg 2014;45(3):e41–5.

158. Lehnert P, Moller CH, Damgaard S, et al. Transit-time flow measurement as a predictor of coronary bypass graft failure at one year angiographic follow-up. J Card Surg 2015;30(1):47–52.

159. Niclauss L. Techniques and standards in intraoperative graft verification by transit time flow measurement after coronary artery bypass graft surgery: a critical review. Eur J Cardiothorac Surg 2017;51(1):26–33.

160. Jokinen JJ, Werkkala K, Vainikka T, et al. Clinical value of intra-operative transit-time flow measurement for coronary artery bypass grafting: a prospective angiography-controlled study. Eur J Cardiothorac Surg 2011;39(6):918–23.

161. Head SJ, Milojevic M, Daemen J, et al. Stroke rates following surgical versus percutaneous coronary revascularization. J Am Coll Cardiol 2018; 72(4):386–98.

162. Afilalo J, Rasti M, Ohayon SM, et al. Off-pump vs. on-pump coronary artery bypass surgery: an updated meta-analysis and meta-regression of randomized trials. Eur Heart J 2012;33(10):1257–67.

163. Deppe AC, Arbash W, Kuhn EW, et al. Current evidence of coronary artery bypass grafting off-pump versus on-pump: a systematic review with meta-analysis of over 16,900 patients investigated in randomized controlled trialsdagger. Eur J Cardiothorac Surg 2016;49(4):1031–41 [discussion: 1041].

164. Kowalewski M, Pawliszak W, Malvindi PG, et al. Off-pump coronary artery bypass grafting improves short-term outcomes in high-risk patients compared with on-pump coronary artery bypass grafting: meta-analysis. J Thorac Cardiovasc Surg 2016;151(1):60–77.e1-58.

165. Borgermann J, Hakim K, Renner A, et al. Clampless off-pump versus conventional coronary artery revascularization: a propensity score analysis of 788 patients. Circulation 2012;126(11 Suppl 1): S176–82.

166. Guerrieri Wolf L, Abu-Omar Y, Choudhary BP, et al. Gaseous and solid cerebral microembolization during proximal aortic anastomoses in off-pump coronary surgery: the effect of an aortic side-biting clamp and two clampless devices. J Thorac Cardiovasc Surg 2007;133(2):485–93.

167. El Zayat H, Puskas JD, Hwang S, et al. Avoiding the clamp during off-pump coronary artery bypass reduces cerebral embolic events: results of a prospective randomized trial. Interact Cardiovasc Thorac Surg 2012;14(1):12–6.

168. Misfeld M, Brereton RJ, Sweetman EA, et al. Neurologic complications after off-pump coronary artery bypass grafting with and without aortic manipulation: meta-analysis of 11,398 cases from 8 studies. J Thorac Cardiovasc Surg 2011;142(2): e11–7.

169. Zhao DF, Edelman JJ, Seco M, et al. Coronary artery bypass grafting with and without manipulation of the ascending aorta: a network meta-analysis. J Am Coll Cardiol 2017;69(8):924–36.

170. Ozatik MA, Gol MK, Fansa I, et al. Risk factors for stroke following coronary artery bypass operations. J Card Surg 2005;20(1):52–7.

171. Rosenberger P, Shernan SK, Loffler M, et al. The influence of epiaortic ultrasonography on intraoperative surgical management in 6051 cardiac surgical patients. Ann Thorac Surg 2008;85(2):548–53.

172. Konety SH, Rosenthal GE, Vaughan-Sarrazin MS. Surgical volume and outcomes of off-pump coronary artery bypass graft surgery: does it matter? J Thorac Cardiovasc Surg 2009;137(5):1116–23.e1.

173. Head SJ, Borgermann J, Osnabrugge RL, et al. Coronary artery bypass grafting: part 2–optimizing outcomes and future prospects. Eur Heart J 2013;34(37):2873–86.

174. Holzhey DM, Cornely JP, Rastan AJ, et al. Review of a 13-year single-center experience with minimally invasive direct coronary artery bypass as the primary surgical treatment of coronary artery disease. Heart Surg Forum 2012;15(2):E61–8.

175. Raja SG, Benedetto U, Alkizwini E, et al, Harefield Cardiac Outcomes Research Group. Propensity score adjusted comparison of MIDCAB versus full sternotomy left anterior descending artery revascularization. Innovations (Phila) 2015;10(3): 174–8.

176. Diegeler A, Walther T, Metz S, et al. Comparison of MIDCAP versus conventional CABG surgery regarding pain and quality of life. Heart Surg Forum 1999;2(4):290–5 [discussion: 295–6].

177. Groh MA, Sutherland SE, Burton HG 3rd, et al. Port-access coronary artery bypass grafting: technique and comparative results. Ann Thorac Surg 1999;68(4):1506–8.

178. Lapierre H, Chan V, Sohmer B, et al. Minimally invasive coronary artery bypass grafting via a small thoracotomy versus off-pump: a case-matched study. Eur J Cardiothorac Surg 2011;40(4):804–10.

179. Thiele H, Neumann-Schniedewind P, Jacobs S, et al. Randomized comparison of minimally invasive direct coronary artery bypass surgery versus sirolimus-eluting stenting in isolated proximal

left anterior descending coronary artery stenosis. J Am Coll Cardiol 2009;53(25):2324–31.

180. Blazek S, Rossbach C, Borger MA, et al. Comparison of sirolimus-eluting stenting with minimally invasive bypass surgery for stenosis of the left anterior descending coronary artery: 7-year follow-up of a randomized trial. JACC Cardiovasc Interv 2015;8(1 Pt A):30–8.

181. Deppe AC, Liakopoulos OJ, Kuhn EW, et al. Minimally invasive direct coronary bypass grafting versus percutaneous coronary intervention for single-vessel disease: a meta-analysis of 2885 patients. Eur J Cardiothorac Surg 2015;47(3):397–406 [discussion: 406].

182. Wang XW, Qu C, Huang C, et al. Minimally invasive direct coronary bypass compared with percutaneous coronary intervention for left anterior descending artery disease: a meta-analysis. J Cardiothorac Surg 2016;11(1):125.

183. Gasior M, Zembala MO, Tajstra M, et al. Hybrid revascularization for multivessel coronary artery disease. JACC Cardiovasc Interv 2014;7(11): 1277–83.

184. Bonatti JO, Zimrin D, Lehr EJ, et al. Hybrid coronary revascularization using robotic totally endoscopic surgery: perioperative outcomes and 5-year results. Ann Thorac Surg 2012;94(6):1920–6 [discussion: 1926].

185. Shen L, Hu S, Wang H, et al. One-stop hybrid coronary revascularization versus coronary artery bypass grafting and percutaneous coronary intervention for the treatment of multivessel coronary artery disease: 3-year follow-up results from a single institution. J Am Coll Cardiol 2013;61(25): 2525–33.

186. Harskamp RE, Bonatti JO, Zhao DX, et al. Standardizing definitions for hybrid coronary revascularization. J Thorac Cardiovasc Surg 2014;147(2): 556–60.

187. Tajstra M, Hrapkowicz T, Hawranek M, et al. Hybrid coronary revascularization in selected patients with multivessel disease: 5-year clinical outcomes of the prospective randomized pilot study. JACC Cardiovasc Interv 2018;11(9):847–52.

188. Modrau IS, Holm NR, Maeng M, et al. One-year clinical and angiographic results of hybrid coronary revascularization. J Thorac Cardiovasc Surg 2015;150(5):1181–6.

189. Harskamp RE, Brennan JM, Xian Y, et al. Practice patterns and clinical outcomes after hybrid coronary revascularization in the United States: an analysis from the society of thoracic surgeons adult cardiac database. Circulation 2014;130(11): 872–9.

190. Puskas JD, Halkos ME, DeRose JJ, et al. Hybrid coronary revascularization for the treatment of multivessel coronary artery disease: a multicenter

observational study. J Am Coll Cardiol 2016; 68(4):356–65.

191. Bonatti J, Schachner T, Bonaros N, et al. Robotically assisted totally endoscopic coronary bypass surgery. Circulation 2011;124(2):236–44.

192. Pinho-Gomes AC, Azevedo L, Ahn JM, et al. Compliance with guideline-directed medical therapy in contemporary coronary revascularization trials. J Am Coll Cardiol 2018;71(6):591–602.

193. Kapur A, Hall RJ, Malik IS, et al. Randomized comparison of percutaneous coronary intervention with coronary artery bypass grafting in diabetic patients. 1-year results of the CARDia (Coronary Artery Revascularization in Diabetes) trial. J Am Coll Cardiol 2010;55(5):432–40.

194. Farkouh ME, Domanski M, Sleeper LA, et al. Strategies for multivessel revascularization in patients with diabetes. N Engl J Med 2012;367(25):2375–84.

195. Kamalesh M, Sharp TG, Tang XC, et al. Percutaneous coronary intervention versus coronary bypass surgery in United States veterans with diabetes. J Am Coll Cardiol 2013;61(8):808–16.

196. Park SJ, Ahn JM, Kim YH, et al. Trial of everolimus-eluting stents or bypass surgery for coronary disease. N Engl J Med 2015;372(13):1204–12.

197. Ahn JM, Roh JH, Kim YH, et al. Randomized trial of stents versus bypass surgery for left main coronary artery disease: 5-year outcomes of the PRECOMBAT Study. J Am Coll Cardiol 2015;65(20): 2198–206.

198. Hakeem A, Garg N, Bhatti S, et al. Effectiveness of percutaneous coronary intervention with drug-eluting stents compared with bypass surgery in diabetics with multivessel coronary disease: comprehensive systematic review and meta-analysis of randomized clinical data. J Am Heart Assoc 2013;2(4):e000354.

199. Al Ali J, Franck C, Filion KB, et al. Coronary artery bypass graft surgery versus percutaneous coronary intervention with first-generation drug-eluting stents: a meta-analysis of randomized controlled trials. JACC Cardiovasc Interv 2014; 7(5):497–506.

200. Sipahi I, Akay MH, Dagdelen S, et al. Coronary artery bypass grafting vs percutaneous coronary intervention and long-term mortality and morbidity in multivessel disease: meta-analysis of randomized clinical trials of the arterial grafting and stenting era. JAMA Intern Med 2014;174(2): 223–30.

201. Lim JY, Deo SV, Kim WS, et al. Drug-eluting stents versus coronary artery bypass grafting in diabetic patients with multi-vessel disease: a meta-analysis. Heart Lung Circ 2014;23(8):717–25.

202. D'Ascenzo F, Barbero U, Moretti C, et al. Percutaneous coronary intervention versus coronary

artery bypass graft for stable angina: meta-regression of randomized trials. Contemp Clin Trials 2014;38(1):51–8.

203. Fanari Z, Weiss SA, Zhang W, et al. Comparison of percutaneous coronary intervention with drug eluting stents versus coronary artery bypass grafting in patients with multivessel coronary artery disease: Meta-analysis of six randomized controlled trials. Cardiovasc Revasc Med 2015; 16(2):70–7.

204. Zimarino M, Ricci F, Romanello M, et al. Complete myocardial revascularization confers a larger clinical benefit when performed with state-of-the-art techniques in high-risk patients with multivessel coronary artery disease: A meta-analysis of randomized and observational studies. Catheter Cardiovasc Interv 2016;87(1):3–12.

205. Benedetto U, Gaudino M, Ng C, et al. Coronary surgery is superior to drug eluting stents in multivessel disease. Systematic review and meta-analysis of contemporary randomized controlled trials. Int J Cardiol 2016;210:19–24.

206. Lee CW, Ahn JM, Cavalcante R, et al. Coronary artery bypass surgery versus drug-eluting stent implantation for left main or multivessel coronary artery disease: a meta-analysis of individual patient data. JACC Cardiovasc Interv 2016;9(24): 2481–9.

Percutaneous Coronary Intervention for the Treatment of Spontaneous Coronary Artery Dissection

Anthony Main, MD[a],
Jacqueline Saw, MD, FRCPC, FSCAI[b],*

KEYWORDS

- Spontaneous coronary artery dissection • Percutaneous coronary intervention
- Myocardial infarction • Cutting balloon • Stent

KEY POINTS

- Conservative therapy is preferred for SCAD patients unless there is high-risk features of ongoing ischemia, left main dissection, or hemodynamic or electrical instability.
- PCI options include cutting balloon fenestration, angioplasty alone, stenting edges before the middle, and bioabsorbable stents.
- PCI is preferred over CABG if technically feasible.

INTRODUCTION

Spontaneous coronary artery dissection (SCAD) is an important and increasingly recognized cause of myocardial infarction (MI) in young to middle-aged women.[1,2] SCAD is defined as a nontraumatic, noniatrogenic, and nonatherosclerotic separation of the coronary arterial wall by an intramural hematoma (IMH), creating a false lumen, which then compresses the true lumen, causing myocardial ischemia or infarction.[1] The separation can occur between the intima, media, or adventitia and can originate from an intimal tear leading to dissection into the arterial wall or may result from spontaneous bleeding from ruptured vasa vasorum without intimal tear.[1,3] The pathophysiology of SCAD remains incompletely understood, but there is often an underlying arteriopathy that weakens the arterial wall, with associated additional physical, emotional, and/or hormonal stressors that trigger the dissection.[4]

Although randomized, controlled trials regarding the optimal management strategy for SCAD are lacking, observational studies and expert consensus suggest that a conservative treatment approach is preferred in the absence of high-risk features.[2,5–7] This finding is based primarily on the observations that dissected artery segments heal over time and that revascularization is associated with high failure and complication rates. Although the majority of patients can be managed conservatively, patients with ongoing ischemia, left main dissection, electrical or hemodynamic instability, or other high-risk features should be considered for revascularization. To date, few reports have been published in the literature regarding techniques for the percutaneous management of SCAD.

The purpose of this review is to discuss the basis for conservative versus invasive management of SCAD, summarize the indications for revascularization, to review the challenges of

---

[a] Division of Cardiology, Foothills Medical Centre, University of Calgary, 1403 29 St NW, Calgary, AB T2N 2T9, Canada; [b] Interventional Cardiology, Division of Cardiology, Vancouver General Hospital, University of British Columbia, 2775 Laurel Street, Level 9, Vancouver, British Columbia V5Z1M9, Canada
* Corresponding author.
E-mail address: jsaw@mail.ubc.ca

Intervent Cardiol Clin 8 (2019) 199–208
https://doi.org/10.1016/j.iccl.2018.11.008
2211-7458/19/© 2018 Elsevier Inc. All rights reserved.

percutaneous coronary intervention (PCI) with SCAD, and to discuss the technical aspects for PCI with SCAD.

OUTCOMES WITH CONSERVATIVE AND INVASIVE MANAGEMENT OF SPONTANEOUS CORONARY ARTERY DISSECTION

The management of MI owing to atherosclerotic coronary artery disease differs significantly than that owing to SCAD. Clinical guidelines recommend an early invasive strategy and revascularization over conservative therapy for acute coronary syndrome presentations with coronary artery disease,[8] whereas conservative therapy for SCAD is preferred over revascularization, based on the natural tendency for spontaneous arterial healing and the risks of PCI with SCAD.

Several small cases series had reported spontaneous angiographic healing in the majority of dissected segments (73%–97% of cases) where repeat coronary angiograms were performed for conservatively managed patients.[1,2,9,10] In the absence of instrumentation with angioplasty or stenting, the natural history of SCAD seems to be spontaneous healing with gradual resorption of the IMH, and eventual tacking up of the dissection flap against deeper arterial walls over days to weeks. There seems to be some time latency for arterial healing to occur. Early resorption of IMH had been described to start within days of the dissection on optical coherence tomography (OCT),[11] and complete angiographic healing have been reported to occur within 4 to 6 weeks.[9]

PCI of SCAD is associated with relatively low technical success rates and high complication rates.[1,2,6,9] In the large Vancouver cohort of 327 patients with SCAD, 54 underwent PCI; 43.1% of procedures were deemed successful, 25.9% were partially successful, and 31.0% were unsuccessful.[12] In the Mayo Clinic 189-patient series, PCI failure was reported in 53%.[2] In our prior 168-patient Vancouver cohort, successful or partially successful PCI was achieved in 64%, with 57% having extension of dissections during PCI, 12% requiring urgent coronary artery bypass (CABG) surgery, and 6% had stent thrombosis; long-term durable results was achieved in only 30%.[9] In the Italian 134-patient series, unsuccessful PCI was reported in 27.5% of patients (with stent thrombosis occurring in 5%). Patients treated conservatively had a lower rate of in-hospital major cardiac adverse events compared with those treated with revascularization (3.8% vs 16.1%; P = .028).[6] Other reported

series are much smaller and the results are summarized in Table 1.

Patients managed conservatively should be monitored in-hospital for signs of extension of dissection, which can result in recurrent MI or unplanned revascularization. The reported incidences of in-hospital recurrent MI, need for urgent revascularization, or other major adverse events are between 5% and 10%.[6,9,13] In our 168-patient Vancouver cohort, 134 patients (79.8%) were managed conservatively and 3 of these patients (1.7%) subsequently required revascularization for SCAD extension.[9] In the updated 327-patient Vancouver cohort, 272 patients (83.2%) were treated conservatively, and subsequently 3.3% had extension of dissection and required in-hospital revascularization (2.2% with PCI, 1.1% with CABG).[12] In the Mayo Clinic cohort, 9 of 94 patients (9.6%) who were managed conservatively had progression of their SCAD and required revascularization.[2] In the series by Alfonso and associates,[7] of the 45 patients with SCAD who were managed conservatively, 16 (35.6%) required revascularization during their initial hospitalization and 2 required revascularization at follow-up.

Expert consensus statements recommend monitoring in-hospital for 3 to 5 days.[5,14] Medical therapy should be instituted in the form of beta-blockade to decrease arterial shear stress, and dual antiplatelet therapy (DAPT; typically aspirin and clopidogrel) should be administered for acute treatment.[1] Angiotensin-converting enzyme inhibitors or angiotensin receptor blockers should be administered for those with left ventricular dysfunction, and statins for those with underlying dyslipidemia.[1] In general, unfractionated heparin, glycoprotein IIb/IIIa inhibitors, oral anticoagulants, and thrombolytics should be avoided in cases of SCAD to prevent extension of the IMH.

INDICATIONS FOR REVASCULARIZATION

Although conservative therapy is the preferred treatment for SCAD and can be applied to the majority of clinically stable patients, there are clinical situations in which revascularization should be pursued. Patients with clinical evidence of ongoing ischemia (eg, electrocardiographic changes, ischemic chest pain), cardiogenic shock, sustained ventricular arrhythmias, and left main dissection, who have technically feasible anatomy for PCI, should typically undergo percutaneous revascularization. In cases where PCI is not deemed feasible or fails, then CABG should be considered.

Table 1
Outcomes with percutaneous in spontaneous coronary artery dissection studies

Studies, Year	N	Age (y)	Women (%)	ACS (%)	STEMI (%)	NSTEMI (%)	Revascularization (%)	PCI (%)	PCI Success (%)
Saw et al,[12] 2017	327	52.5 ± 9.6	90.8	100	25.7	74.3	18.7	16.5	69.0
Nakashimi et al,[20] 2016	63	46.0 ± 10.0	94.9	100	87.0	13.0	55.6	54.0	91.0
Rashid et al,[23] 2016	21	53.3 ± 8.8	95.2	100	34.8	56.5	28.6	28.6	66.7
Roura et al,[24] 2016	34	47.0 ± 12.0	94.1	100	55.0	45.0	23.5	23.5	75.0
Rogowski et al,[10] 2017	64	53.0 ± 11.2	94.0	100	69.0	30.0	12.5	10.9	66.7
Lettieri et al,[6] 2015	134	52.0 ± 11.0	81.0	93.0	49.2	40.3	42.0	38.3	72.5
Tweet et al,[2] 2014	189	44.0 ± 9.0	92.0	100	37.0	63.0	50.3	47.1	47.0
Saw et al,[9] 2014	168	52.1 ± 9.2	92.3	100	26.1	73.9	20.2	16.7	63.6
Alfonso et al,[7] 2012	27	53.0 ± 11.0	85.0	85.0	52.0	33.0	55.6	55.6	80.0

Abbreviations: NSTEMI, non–ST-segment elevation myocardial infarction; PCI, proportion who underwent percutaneous coronary intervention; Revascularization, proportion who underwent revascularization; STEMI, ST-segment elevation myocardial infarction.

Patients with SCAD of the left main artery should generally be considered for revascularization, preferably with CABG if the dissection is extensive. PCI may be considered for left main dissection if emergency CABG is not available, in patients who are hemodynamically/electrically unstable and unlikely to survive with the delay to emergency CABG, and those with technically

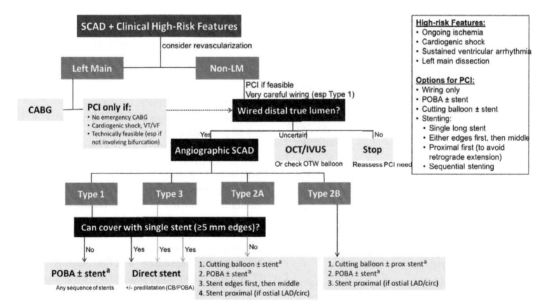

Fig. 1. Percutaneous coronary intervention (PCI) algorithm. [a] Can avoid stenting especially if normal flow + no residual dissection. CABG, coronary artery bypass grafting; IVUS, intravascular ultrasound; LAD, left anterior descending; OCT, optical coherence tomography; OTW, over the wire; POBA, plain old balloon angioplasty; VT/VF, ventricular tachycardia/ventricular fibrillation. (*Reprinted from* EuroIntervention 14(13), Saw J. Natural history of spontaneous coronary artery dissection: to stent or not to stent?, 1353–6; 2019; with permission from Europa Digital & Publishing.)

feasible anatomy (especially if not involving distal left main bifurcation; Fig. 1).

The American Heart Association Scientific Statement for SCAD recommended that patients with active/ongoing ischemia or hemodynamic instability should undergo PCI (if technically feasible) or urgent CABG, while acknowledging that such decisions must be individualized and based on the expertise of local operators. In patients with left main dissection or severe proximal 2-vessel disease who are clinically stable (ie, no ongoing ischemia or hemodynamic compromise), CABG may be considered; however, conservative therapy may also be reasonable, although this finding is based on anecdotal experience and has not been studied.[5]

CHALLENGES OF PERCUTANEOUS CORONARY INTERVENTION

PCI for SCAD can be technically challenging and is associated with high failure rates and risk of complications (see Table 1).[1] In the Mayo clinic 189-patient series, only 47% of PCI had procedural success.[2] In the Italian cohort, successful PCI was achieved in 72.5% of patients, with 9% requiring CABG and 5% developing stent thrombosis.[6] In the Vancouver 168-patient cohort, successful or partially successful PCI was accomplished in 64% of patients, with extension of dissection occurring in 57%, need for urgent CABG in 12%, and stent thrombosis in 6%.[9]

There are multiple challenges associated with PCI of SCAD (Box 1). Importantly, there is a

---

Box 1
Challenges with percutaneous coronary intervention in patients with spontaneous coronary artery dissection

1. Risk of iatrogenic catheter-induced coronary artery dissection

2. Difficulty advancing coronary wire into the true lumen

3. Extending intimal dissection or intramural hematoma with wiring, angioplasty or stenting

4. Dissection extending into distal arteries too small for stenting

5. Extensive dissections requiring long stents (restenosis risk) if inadequate angioplasty results

6. Resorption of intramural hematoma causing stent malapposition and risk of stent thrombosis

---

significant risk of iatrogenic catheter-induced coronary artery dissection, given the increased fragility of the coronary arteries in patients with SCAD.[15,16] Catheter manipulation and contrast injections must be performed carefully and meticulously when SCAD is suspected. The overall incidence of catheter-induced iatrogenic dissections during routine coronary angiography is uncommon, occurring in less than 0.2% of coronary angiograms.[16] However, we have observed that iatrogenic dissections are more common during coronary angiography in the SCAD population. In our report of 211 prospectively followed patients with nonatherosclerotic SCAD, there were 348 coronary angiograms performed, of which 12 cases of iatrogenic dissection occurred (incidence, 3.4%).[15] Of these iatrogenic dissections, the incidence during diagnostic angiography was 2.0%, and incidence during ad hoc PCI was 14.3%. Nearly all patients (11/12) with iatrogenic dissections required treatment with PCI. Patients who had iatrogenic dissections had a higher proportion of guide catheter usage, deep catheter engagement, and radial artery access. Furthermore, patients with iatrogenic dissections during angiography for their SCAD had higher in-hospital major adverse cardiac events (25.0% vs 5.5%; $P = .036$) compared with other patients with SCAD without iatrogenic dissections.[15]

Wiring dissected lesions can be challenging because there may be difficulty advancing the coronary guidewire into the true lumen, especially in cases of type 1 SCAD, where there is evident intimal disruption.[17] However, angioplasty or stenting of SCAD lesions necessitates wiring into the distal true lumen. Failure to wire into the distal true lumen typically requires aborting the procedure.

Another challenge with PCI for SCAD is the risk of propagation of dissection or IMH with wiring, balloon angioplasty, or stenting. The IMH can propagate anterogradely or retrogradely with any instrumentation, extending the dissection and resulting in the need for additional stents and can worsen distal blood flow. SCAD can also frequently extend into small distal vessels, including to the apical tip of the arteries, which are too small and distal to be treated with stents. Dissected arterial segments with SCAD are often quite extensive, requiring multiple and long stents, which can increase the risk of restenosis and stent thrombosis. Furthermore, the natural history of SCAD includes resorption of IMH over time, which can lead to late stent malapposition that may increase the risk of late stent thrombosis. Lempereur and colleagues[11]

Box 2
Percutaneous coronary intervention strategy options for spontaneous coronary artery dissection described in the literature

1. Balloon angioplasty at minimal pressures to restore blood flow

2. Cutting balloon angioplasty to fenestrate the intima allowing decompression of intramural hematoma from false lumen into true lumen, with or without additional stenting

3. Use of longer stents to cover both edges of dissections by less than 5 mm to decrease the probability of intramural hematoma propagation

4. Stenting the distal and proximal ends of the dissection with short stents before covering the middle of the dissection to prevent intramural hematoma propagation

5. Focal stenting of proximal segment of dissection (or just proximal to the dissection) to prevent proximal extension of intramural hematoma

6. Use of bioabsorbable stents (if available) when long stents are required

described the appearance of stent malapposition on OCT at various stages after SCAD with IMH resorption.

SUGGESTED PERCUTANEOUS CORONARY INTERVENTION STRATEGY WITH SPONTANEOUS CORONARY ARTERY DISSECTION

Given the technical challenges and high failure rates associated with PCI of SCAD, several different and less conventional techniques have been described in the literature (Box 2).[1,18–22] These techniques include the preferential use of angioplasty balloons (including cutting balloon) to improve distal coronary artery perfusion and avoiding the use of long stents that may have increase the subsequent risks of malapposition, stent thrombosis, and restenosis. None of these techniques have been tested in randomized, controlled trials or their outcomes reported in long-term clinical studies. Given that the pathophysiology of SCAD primarily involves IMH in the false lumen compressing the true lumen, the novel use of a cutting balloon to fenestrate the intimal-medial wall to allow decompression of the false lumen is appealing and may circumvent the use of long stents.

Currently available options for PCI with SCAD include (see Fig. 1) (1) wiring only (if flow normalized with wiring alone, or procedure aborted if unable to get into distal true lumen), (2) plain old balloon angioplasty (POBA) with or without additional stenting, (3) cutting balloon fenestration with or without additional stenting, and (4) stenting with various approaches (direct single long stent, stenting either edges first before the middle, stenting proximal edge to avoid retrograde extensions, or sequential stenting from proximal to distal or distal to proximal).

When the decision is made to perform PCI in the setting of SCAD, the operator must proceed with meticulous care and technique to avoid complications. Careful guide catheter engagement and manipulation and cautious and gentle injection of contrast are essential to avoid iatrogenic dissection. The operator should consider using femoral arterial access preferentially, especially if coaxial guide catheter engagement cannot be achieved with the radial approach. The next critical step is careful wiring of the dissected artery, taking care to navigate into the true lumen, especially in the setting of type 1 angiographic SCAD (where intimal dissection is clearly evident; see Fig. 1). The coronary wire needs to be advanced into the distal true lumen before further interventional steps can be taken. If the operator is uncertain about the position of the guidewire relative to the true lumen, intracoronary imaging with either intravascular ultrasound examination or OCT can be helpful. Alternatively, injection through an over-the-wire coronary balloon or microcatheter can be performed to confirm position within the distal true lumen. If the operator is unable to enter into the distal true lumen, the performance of PCI should be reconsidered. At this point, the options are to (1) abort and switch to conservative therapy (especially if ischemia is relieved, and patient is hemodynamically stable), (2) refer for urgent CABG (if there is ongoing ischemia, especially if dissection involves a proximal vessel that jeopardizes a large proportion of myocardium), and (3) step-up to advanced techniques to navigate into the true lumen (eg, the subintimal tracking and reentry technique).

When the coronary guidewire can be successfully navigated into the distal true lumen, we suggest tailoring the decision for angioplasty/stenting according to the angiographic subtypes (see Fig. 1; Figs. 2–5). Type 1 angiographic SCAD describes the presence of contrast dye staining of arterial wall with multiple radiolucent lumen. Type 2 angiographic SCAD describes the appearance of long diffuse narrowing; variant 2A has the appearance of normal arterial segments

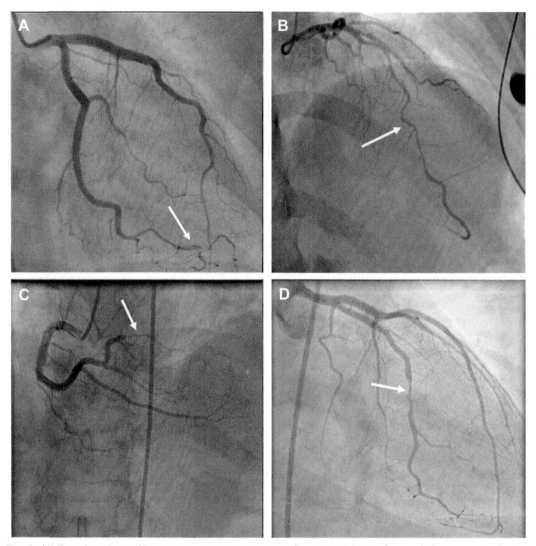

Fig. 2. (A) Type 1 angiographic spontaneous coronary artery dissection (SCAD) of second obtuse marginal artery (*arrow* showing multiple radiolucent lumen). (B) Type 2A angiographic SCAD of the mid to distal left anterior descending (*arrow* showing long diffuse narrowing between normal bordering arterial segments). (C) Type 2B angiographic SCAD of right posterolateral artery (*arrow* showing long diffuse narrowing extending to distal tip of vessel). (D) Type 3 angiographic SCAD of ramus artery (*arrow* showing tubular narrowing).

proximal and distal to the dissection, whereas variant 2B describes the appearance of dissection that extends to the distal tip of the artery. Type 3 angiographic SCAD describes focal or tubular stenosis that mimics atherosclerosis and typically requires OCT or intravascular ultrasound examination to demonstrate the presence of IMH or a double lumen.[2,9,10]

For angiographic SCAD types 1, 2A, or 3, if the dissection can be covered with a single stent, including covering 5 mm or more of normal segments at both edges of the dissection, then direct stenting with a single long stent is the most straightforward strategy. The diameter of the stent must be sized optimally with

either with intracoronary imaging or balloon sizing and the length of the stent should be at least 10 mm longer than the length of the dissection (to accommodate the suggested ≥5-mm of coverage on both ends of the dissection). If the SCAD segment cannot be covered by a single stent, we recommend POBA with or without stenting for type 1 SCAD lesions. For type 2A SCAD lesions that cannot be covered by a single long stent, there are several potential approaches in descending order of preference (see Fig. 1): (1) cutting balloon angioplasty with or without stenting, (2) POBA with or without stenting, (3) stent either edges first before stenting the middle, or (4) stent proximal

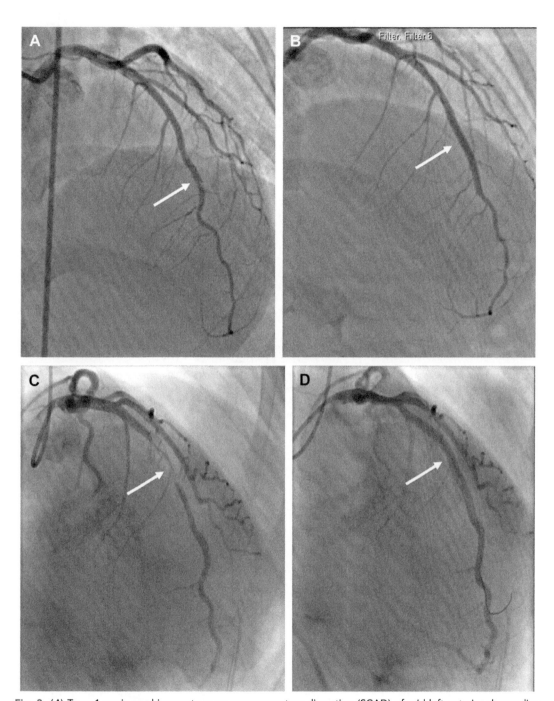

Fig. 3. (A) Type 1 angiographic spontaneous coronary artery dissection (SCAD) of mid left anterior descending (LAD) artery (*arrow*). (B) Long stent for type 1 lesion in A (*arrow*). (C) Type 2A angiographic SCAD of the mid LAD (*arrow*). (D) Long stent for the type 2A lesion in C (*arrow*).

first (especially for ostial left anterior descending or circumflex artery SCAD). After POBA or cutting balloon angioplasty, if coronary flow is normalized (TIMI-3) or if no residual dissection is evident, stenting may be avoided.

For angiographic type 2B SCAD, because the dissection extends into the apical segment of the artery, distal stenting is not possible. In this case, cutting balloon angioplasty with or without stenting of the proximal segment is the

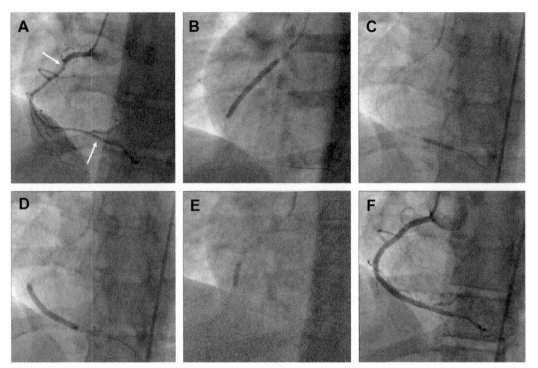

Fig. 4. (*A*) Type 2A angiographic spontaneous coronary artery dissection (SCAD) from the proximal right coronary artery (RCA) to posterior descending artery (PDA; between *arrows*). (*B*) Long stent in the proximal RCA. (*C*) Distal stent into PDA. (*D*) Long stent in the mid RCA. (*E*) Additional short stent in the mid RCA. (*F*) Final angiogram showing results from stenting edges first before the middle.

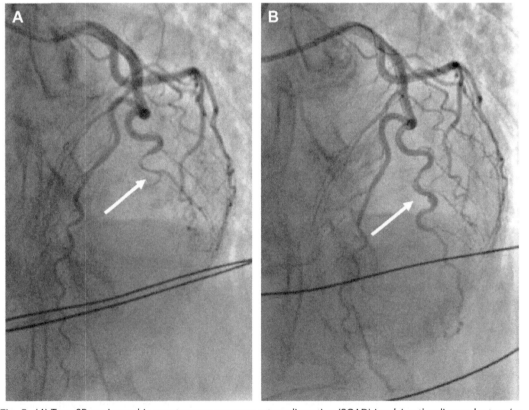

Fig. 5. (*A*) Type 2B angiographic spontaneous coronary artery dissection (SCAD) involving the diagonal artery (*arrow*). (*B*) After cutting balloon angioplasty with final TIMI-3 flow.

preferred strategy. Alternatively, POBA with or without stenting can be pursued, or stenting the proximal dissection (especially if ostial left anterior descending or circumflex artery SCAD; see Fig. 1).

If cutting angioplasty is being considered for SCAD PCI, there are several technical factors that should be considered. Because dissected arteries are fragile and already torn, they are at risk of rupture. Therefore, cutting balloon angioplasty should be done cautiously with small diameter balloons, and we suggest balloon diameter sizing of at least 0.5 mm smaller than the caliber of the vessel being intervened. We recommend inflating to low pressures only (up to 4 atm) to decrease the risk of coronary perforation. Because dissected arteries tend to be tortuous, and cutting balloons tend to be rigid, we suggest using shorter balloons (6 or 10 mm length). The goal of cutting balloon fenestration should be to restore TIMI-3 flow to the artery and in turn alleviate ischemia. This goal may require multiple low-pressure balloon inflations to achieve the desired results. If cutting balloon inflations are insufficient to restore TIMI-3 flow and resolve ischemia, then coronary stents should be deployed. Finally, because cutting balloon angioplasty (especially without stenting) leaves behind disrupted intima, we suggest administering more potent DAPT with aspirin and ticagrelor for at least 1 month until the intima heals, followed by aspirin indefinitely. Scenarios where cutting balloon angioplasty may not be suited include small coronary arteries with diameters of less than 2 mm (because the smallest cutting balloon is 2 mm) and left main dissection. The large caliber left main artery may not be accommodated by available cutting balloon sizes. Furthermore, the potential of creating large dissection flaps in the left main may increase the risk of abrupt vessel occlusion.

After PCI of SCAD lesions, antiplatelet therapy should be continued according to standard post-PCI recommendations.[8] With drug-eluting stent placement, 1 year of DAPT is recommended. For PCI with POBA or cutting balloon angioplasty without stenting, DAPT for at least 1 month is recommended, preferably to 1 year.

SUMMARY

The majority of patients presenting with MI owing to SCAD can be managed conservatively with medical therapy. However, revascularization should be pursued in the presence of high-risk features such as left main dissection, ongoing ischemia, and hemodynamic or electrical instability. Generally PCI is preferred over CABG if technically feasible, except in the setting of left main dissection. However, PCI of SCAD lesions can be technically challenging and is associated with high complication and failure rates. Interventionists should exercise extreme caution and meticulous techniques when performing PCI of SCAD lesions. The novel approach of using cutting balloon to fenestrate and decompress the false lumen is appealing and may avoid the need for long stents. Other percutaneous approaches may also be feasible, and interventionists should be familiar with these various approaches when embarking on SCAD PCI.

REFERENCES

1. Saw J, Mancini GB, Humphries KH. Contemporary review on spontaneous coronary artery dissection. J Am Coll Cardiol 2016;68:297–312.

2. Tweet MS, Eleid MF, Best PJ, et al. Spontaneous coronary artery dissection: revascularization versus conservative therapy. Circ Cardiovasc Interv 2014; 7:777–86.

3. Saw J. Spontaneous coronary artery dissection. Can J Cardiol 2013;29:1027–33.

4. Pretty H. Dissecting aneurysm of coronary artery in a women aged 42. Br Med J 1931;1:667.

5. Hayes SN, Kim ESH, Saw J, et al. Spontaneous coronary artery dissection: current state of the science: a scientific statement from the American Heart Association. Circulation 2018;137:e523–57.

6. Lettieri C, Zavalloni D, Rossini R, et al. Management and long-term prognosis of spontaneous coronary artery dissection. Am J Cardiol 2015;116:66–73.

7. Alfonso F, Paulo M, Lennie V, et al. Spontaneous coronary artery dissection: long-term follow-up of a large series of patients prospectively managed with a "conservative" therapeutic strategy. JACC Cardiovasc Interv 2012;5:1062–70.

8. Amsterdam EA, Wenger NK, Brindis RG, et al. 2014 AHA/ACC guideline for the management of patients with non-ST-elevation acute coronary syndromes: executive summary: a report of the American College of Cardiology/American Heart Association Task Force on practice guidelines. Circulation 2014;130:2354–94.

9. Saw J, Aymong E, Sedlak T, et al. Spontaneous coronary artery dissection: association with predisposing arteriopathies and precipitating stressors and cardiovascular outcomes. Circ Cardiovasc Interv 2014;7:645–55.

10. Rogowski S, Maeder MT, Weilenmann D, et al. Spontaneous coronary artery dissection: angiographic follow-up and long-term clinical outcome in a predominantly medically treated population. Catheter Cardiovasc Interv 2017;89(1):59–68.

11. Lempereur M, Fung A, Saw J. Stent mal-apposition with resorption of intramural hematoma with spontaneous coronary artery dissection. Cardiovasc Diagn Ther 2015;5:323–9.

12. Saw J, Humphries K, Aymong E, et al. Spontaneous coronary artery dissection: clinical outcomes and risk of recurrence. J Am Coll Cardiol 2017;70: 1148–58.

13. Tweet MS, Hayes SN, Pitta SR, et al. Clinical features, management and prognosis of spontaneous coronary artery dissection. Circulation 2012;126: 579–88.

14. Adlam D, Alfonso F, Maas A, et al. European Society of Cardiology, acute cardiovascular care association, SCAD study group: a position paper on spontaneous coronary artery dissection. Eur Heart J 2018;39(36):3353–68.

15. Prakash R, Starovoytov A, Heydari M, et al. Catheter-induced iatrogenic coronary artery dissection in patients with spontaneous coronary artery dissection. JACC Cardiovasc Interv 2016;9:1851–3.

16. Awadalla H, Sabet S, El Sebaie A, et al. Catheter-induced left main dissection incidence, predisposition and therapeutic strategies experience from two sides of the hemisphere. J Invasive Cardiol 2005;17:233–6.

17. Saw J. Coronary angiogram classification of spontaneous coronary artery dissection. Catheter Cardiovasc Interv 2014;84:1115–22.

18. Walsh SJ, Jokhi PP, Saw J. Successful percutaneous management of coronary dissection and extensive intramural haematoma associated with ST elevation MI. Acute Card Care 2008;10:231–3.

19. Watt J, Egred M, Khurana A, et al. 1-year follow-up optical frequency domain imaging of multiple bioresorbable vascular scaffolds for the treatment of spontaneous coronary artery dissection. JACC Cardiovasc Interv 2016;9:389–91.

20. Nakashima T, Noguchi T, Haruta S, et al. Prognostic impact of spontaneous coronary artery dissection in young female patients with acute myocardial infarction: a report from the Angina Pectoris-Myocardial Infarction Multicenter Investigators in Japan. Int J Cardiol 2016;207:341–8.

21. Alfonso F, Bastante T, Garcia-Guimaraes M, et al. Spontaneous coronary artery dissection: new insights into diagnosis and treatment. Coron Artery Dis 2016;27:696–706.

22. Alkhouli M, Cole M, Ling FS. Coronary artery fenestration prior to stenting in spontaneous coronary artery dissection. Catheter Cardiovasc Interv 2015; 88(1):E23–7.

23. Rashid HN, Wong DT, Wijesekera H, et al. Incidence and characterisation of spontaneous coronary artery dissection as a cause of acute coronary syndrome - a single-centre Australian experience. Int J Cardiol 2016;202:336–8.

24. Roura G, Ariza-Sole A, Rodriguez-Caballero IF, et al. Noninvasive follow-up of patients with spontaneous coronary artery dissection with CT angiography. JACC Cardiovasc Imaging 2016;9(7): 896–7.

Periprocedural Myocardial Infarction in Contemporary Practice

David W. Lee, MD*, Matthew A. Cavender, MD, MPH

KEYWORDS

- Myocardial infarction • Percutaneous coronary intervention
- Periprocedural myocardial infarction

KEY POINTS

- Periprocedural myocardial infarction (MI) is associated with an increased risk of mortality and morbidity.
- Periprocedural MI can occur due to side branch occlusion, distal embolization, microvascular obstruction, dissection, or formation of intracoronary thrombus.
- Therapeutic strategies to reduce the risk of periprocedural MI include pretreatment with oral dual antiplatelet therapy, intravenous P2Y12 inhibitors (cangrelor), intravenous glycoprotein IIb/IIIa inhibitors (eptifibatide, abciximab, tirofiban), anticoagulation (heparin, enoxaparin, bivalirudin), and embolic protection devices.

INTRODUCTION

In the contemporary era of interventional cardiology, the risk of in-hospital mortality following percutaneous coronary interventions (PCI) is less than 2%.[1] Despite this low risk of mortality, complications such as periprocedural myocardial infarction (MI) occur during PCI. Approximately 3% to 6% of patients have periprocedural MI following PCI and up to one-third of patients have evidence of procedural myocardial injury.[2–4] Numerous studies have demonstrated that periprocedural MI is associated with an increased risk of morbidity and mortality.[5–21] A thorough understanding of periprocedural MI can help in the identification of patients who are at increased risk and may benefit from strategies designed to mitigate this risk. The objective of this review is to discuss the definitions, prognostic significance, mechanisms, predictors, and preventative strategies for periprocedural MI.

DEFINITIONS OF PERIPROCEDURAL MYOCARDIAL INFARCTION

MI occurs when there is irreversible myocardial injury that results in myocardial death. Although there are multiple ways in which MI can occur, the mechanisms are fundamentally linked by a lack of coronary artery perfusion to the myocardium. Standardized methods to describe coronary artery perfusion have been developed and are well validated. The Thrombolysis in Myocardial Infarction (TIMI) Flow Grade is an objective measure of coronary blood flow that is used in clinical practice and has been used as an endpoint in randomized trials[22] (Table 1). Multiple studies have validated the prognostic significance of TIMI flow following intervention. Patients with TIMI flow less than 3 at the end of case are at considerably higher risk of adverse cardiovascular events.[23,24]

Epicardial blood flow is a good surrogate for myocardial perfusion; however, microvascular

---

Disclosures: Dr D.W. Lee has no relevant disclosures. Dr M.A. Cavender reports relevant research and consulting fees from Chiesi, AstraZeneca, and Merck.
Division of Interventional Cardiology, University of North Carolina, 160 Dental Circle, CB 7075, Chapel Hill, NC 27599, USA
* Corresponding author.
E-mail address: David.Lee@unchealth.unc.edu

Intervent Cardiol Clin 8 (2019) 209–223
https://doi.org/10.1016/j.iccl.2018.12.001
2211-7458/19/© 2018 Elsevier Inc. All rights reserved.

Table 1
Angiographic Grading Scales to assess flow following percutaneous revascularization

Grade	TIMI Flow Grade[22]	TIMI Myocardial Blush Grade[25]
0	Complete occlusion	No apparent tissue-level perfusion (no ground-glass appearance of blush or opacification of the myocardium) in the distribution of the culprit artery
1	Penetration of obstruction by contrast but no distal perfusion	Presence of myocardial blush but no clearance from the microvasculature (blush or a stain was present on the next injection)
2	Perfusion of entire artery but delayed flow	Blush clears slowly (blush is strongly persistent and diminishes minimally or not at all during 3 cardiac cycles of the washout phase)
3	Full perfusion, normal flow	Blush begins to clear during washout (blush is minimally persistent after 3 cardiac cycles of washout)

obstruction can be present even in the presence of adequate epicardial blood flow. The TIMI myocardial perfusion grade (TMP) was developed to quantify angiographic evidence of myocardial perfusion (see Table 1).[25] In the TIMI 10B trial (n = 762), patients with evidence of normal microvascular perfusion (TMP grade 3) had the lowest mortality. There is an inverse relationship between microvascular perfusion and mortality, such that those patients with the lowest TMP have the highest mortality. This relationship is seen even among patients who have TIMI 3 flow in the epicardial infarct artery. Additional risk scores have also been developed, which have used similar grading scales and have also been shown to be associated with cardiovascular events.[26]

Over time, there has been considerable debate regarding the appropriate definition for a periprocedural MI.[27] In the current era, 2 distinct definitions for periprocedural MI are used most frequently, the Fourth Universal definition of MI related to PCI (type 4a MI) and the Society for Cardiovascular Angiography and Interventions (SCAI) definition of clinically relevant MI after PCI.[28,29] Although there are fundamental differences in these definitions, both compare baseline cardiac biomarker values before PCI with cardiac biomarker values following PCI.

In the Fourth Universal Definition, cardiac troponin is the preferred biomarker of myocardial injury and is used for the diagnosis of periprocedural MI (Table 2).[28] In patients with baseline values that are normal (less than 99th percentile of the upper reference limit [URL]), a periprocedural MI is defined as cardiac troponin elevation with values greater than 5x the 99th percentile of the URL within the first 48 hours following PCI.[28] In patients with elevated baseline values that are stable or falling, a periprocedural MI is defined as a cardiac troponin increase of greater than or equal to 20% within the first 48 hours following PCI. In addition to fulfilling the biomarker criteria, patients must have objective evidence of myocardial ischemia defined as at least one of the following: ischemic symptoms for at least 20 minutes, new ST-segment changes that suggest ischemia, new pathologic Q waves, or new left bundle branch block (LBBB) on electrocardiography (ECG), angiographic evidence of the loss of patency of a major coronary artery or a side branch, no reflow or slow flow, or distal embolization, or imaging demonstrating new loss of viable myocardium or new regional wall motion abnormality.

In contrast, the SCAI definition of clinically relevant MI after PCI uses creatine kinase-muscle/brain (CK-MB) rather than cardiac troponin.[29] In addition, this definition relies predominately on biomarker elevation and does not account for patient symptoms in those patients with normal biomarkers at baseline. In patients with normal baseline values or elevated baseline values that are stable or falling, a periprocedural MI is defined as CK-MB elevation with values greater than or equal to 10x the local laboratory upper limit of normal (ULN) or values greater than or equal to 5x ULN with new pathologic Q waves in at least 2 contiguous leads or a new persistent LBBB on ECG, all within the first 48 hours following PCI.[29] In patients without CK-MB measurements and with normal baseline cardiac troponin values or elevated baseline cardiac troponin values that are stable or falling, a periprocedural MI is defined as cardiac troponin

Table 2 Definitions of periprocedural myocardial infarction		
Baseline Cardiac Biomarker Levels	**Fourth Universal Definition of MI (Peri-PCI, Type IVa)**	**SCAI Definition of Clinically Relevant MI after PCI**
Normal	Troponin >5x the 99th percentile of the upper reference limit within the first 48 h following PCI and at least one of the following criteria: • Ischemic symptoms for 20 min • Electrocardiogram with new ST-segment changes that suggest ischemia, new pathologic Q waves, or new left bundle branch block • Angiography with loss of patency of a major coronary artery or a side branch, no reflow or slow flow, or distal embolization • Imaging with new loss of viable myocardium or new regional wall motion abnormality	CK-MB >10 times the upper limit of normal, or CK-MB >5 times the upper limit of normal, with electrocardiogram showing new pathologic Q waves in at least 2 contiguous leads or a new persistent left bundle branch block, within the first 48 h following PCI In patients without CK-MB values: Troponin >70 times the upper limit of normal, or troponin >35 times the upper limit of normal, with electrocardiogram showing new pathologic Q waves in at least 2 contiguous leads or a new persistent left bundle branch block, within the first 48 h following PCI
Elevated (Stable or Falling)	Troponin increase of at least 20% within the first 48 h following PCI and at least one of the following criteria: • Ischemic symptoms for 20 min • Electrocardiogram with new ST-segment changes that suggest ischemia, new pathologic Q waves, or new left bundle branch block • Angiography with loss of patency of a major coronary artery or a side branch, no reflow or slow flow, or distal embolization • Imaging with new loss of viable myocardium or new regional wall motion abnormality	CK-MB >10 times the upper limit of normal, or CK-MB >5 times the upper limit of normal, with electrocardiogram showing new pathologic Q waves in at least 2 contiguous leads or a new persistent left bundle branch block, within the first 48 h following PCI In patients without CK-MB values: Troponin >70 times the upper limit of normal, or troponin >35 times the upper limit of normal, with electrocardiogram showing new pathologic Q waves in at least 2 contiguous leads or a new persistent left bundle branch block, within the first 48 h following PCI
Elevated (Rising)	Not defined	In addition to the above cardiac biomarker criteria: Electrocardiogram with new ST-segment elevation or depression and signs consistent with a clinically relevant MI (ie, sustained hypotension or new-onset or worsening heart failure)

Abbreviations: CK-MB, creatine kinase-muscle/brain; SCAI, society for cardiovascular angiography interventions.
Adapted from Thygesen K, Alpert JS, Jaffe AS, et al. Fourth universal definition of myocardial infarction (2018). J Am Coll Cardiol 2018;72(18):2231–64; and Moussa ID, Klein LW, Shah B, et al. Consideration of a new definition of clinically relevant myocardial infarction after coronary revascularization: an expert consensus document from the Society for Cardiovascular Angiography and Interventions (SCAI). J Am Coll Cardiol 2013;62(17):1567; with permission.

elevation with values greater than or equal to 70x ULN or with values greater than or equal to 35x ULN with new pathologic Q waves in at least 2 contiguous leads or a new persistent LBBB on ECG, all within the first 48 hours following PCI.[29] In patients with elevated baseline CK-MB or cardiac troponin values that are not stable or falling, the respective diagnostic criteria for CK-MB or cardiac troponin elevation must be accompanied with both evidence of new ST-segment elevation or depression on ECG and signs consistent with a clinically relevant MI such as sustained hypotension or new-onset or worsening heart failure.[29]

There are major differences between the 2 definitions of periprocedural MI. First, the WHO Fourth Universal Definition recommends the use of cardiac troponin, whereas the SCAI definition preferentially recommends the use of CK-MB.[28,29] Compared with CK-MB, cardiac troponin is more sensitive and specific for myocardial injury.[30,31] Prior studies have found that troponin is a better marker and can identify acute coronary syndromes in situations in which CK-MB is not elevated.[32] In addition, assays used to measure CK-MB have increased variability, resulting in analytical issues with measurement of CK-MB. For these reasons, there has been decreased clinical utilization of CK-MB for the diagnosis of MI before PCI and troponin should continue to be the preferred biomarker for myocardial injury. Because of differences in the assays, there are differences in interpretation of fold elevations greater than the upper reference limit between CK-MB and troponin. CK-MB elevation has an association with adverse cardiovascular events in the post-PCI setting that is of greater magnitude when compared with a similar fold elevation of troponin.[5-8,10,14-17,33,34] As such, it is possible that using cardiac troponin as the preferred biomarker results in identification of periprocedural biomarker elevations that would not otherwise be detected and the prognostic implications of these events remains unknown.

The second major difference between the Universal and SCAI definitions is with regard to the presence of symptoms. The Universal definition requires additional features of ischemia/infarction such as symptoms, ECG, angiography, or imaging; the SCAI definition is driven by cardiac biomarker elevation except in those with elevated baseline values that are not stable or falling. Such a biomarker-driven definition may cause an increased false-positive rate, given that successful PCI with optimal stent implantation can also be associated with increased

biomarker values.[35] Moreover, coexisting disease processes that are not related to PCI such as severity of coronary artery disease, heart failure, or arrhythmias can also be associated with increased biomarker values.

Third, although the Universal definition does not address patients with elevated baseline troponin values that are not stable or falling, the SCAI definition clarifies that these patients need additional criteria in order to be diagnosed with periprocedural MI. Because of these major differences, these definitions can be difficult to reconcile in the clinical and research settings. Further investigation is needed to determine the most appropriate definition for MI and to understand how each definition affects prevalence and case-fatality rates associated with periprocedural MI.

PROGNOSTIC SIGNIFICANCE OF PERIPROCEDURAL MYOCARDIAL INFARCTION

There is a clear relationship between elevation in cardiac biomarkers and increased risk of future cardiovascular events. However, the level at which biomarkers elevation is representative of those patients at highest risk versus those cardiovascular events that are a direct result of MI related to the revascularization remains a point of debate. There is a heterogeneous evidence base for the prognostic significance of periprocedural MI. This is largely due to significant variation in study designs, study time periods, PCI strategies, and the definitions of periprocedural MI used by investigators.

Numerous retrospective studies and meta-analyses have demonstrated that post-PCI CK-MB elevation of varying magnitude is associated with increased short-term and long-term mortality, MI, and revascularization.[5-11] Several retrospective studies described this association as a dose-response relationship with higher mortality and morbidity rates seen in patients with higher post-PCI CK-MB elevations, especially in those with CK-MB values greater than 5x ULN.[5,7-9] However, post hoc and pooled analyses of prospective clinical trials failed to demonstrate such robust associations.[33,36] Analyses of 2 large registries highlighted that post-PCI CK-MB values greater than 10 times the upper limit of normal were significantly associated with increased 1-year mortality, a finding that contributed to the formulation of the SCAI definition.[12,13,29] Although some studies have not shown a relationship between elevations in cardiac troponin following PCI and long-term outcomes,[6,10,37,38] most studies have found post-PCI cardiac troponin elevations to be associated with worse outcomes.[14–19,39]

Contemporary large-scale studies have provided robust evidence for the risk of short- and long-term mortality associated with both the Universal and SCAI definitions of periprocedural MI. In a post hoc analysis of the Cangrelor versus Standard Therapy to Achieve Optimal Management of Platelet Inhibition (CHAMPION PHOENIX) trial, a study that randomized 11,145 patients undergoing PCI to cangrelor or clopidogrel, the 30-day mortality risk in patients who fulfilled the SCAI definition of periprocedural MI was significantly elevated (odds ratio [OR] 8.85, 95% confidence interval [CI] 4.29–18.25) as was that among patients who fulfilled the criteria for Universal Type 4a MI (OR 4.6, 95% CI 2.49–8.51) (Fig. 1).[21] In a post hoc analysis of the Early Glycoprotein IIb/IIIa Inhibition in Non-ST-Segment Elevation Acute Coronary Syndrome (EARLY ACS) trial and the Thrombin Receptor Antagonist for Clinical Event Reduction in Acute Coronary Syndrome (TRACER) trial, the hazard ratio (HR) for 1-year mortality was 1.96 (95% CI 1.24–3.10) in patients who fulfilled the criteria for the Universal Third Universal definition of periprocedural MI and 2.79 (95% CI 1.69–4.58) in those meeting the SCAI definition

of periprocedural MI.[20] Finally, a prospective registry of 4514 patients who underwent PCI from 2003 to 2013 demonstrated that patients with the Third Universal Definition of periprocedural MI had a 5-year mortality rate of 12.7%, compared with 8.5% in those without periprocedural MI, with an adjusted HR for mortality of 1.63.[2] In the same study, patients with the SCAI definition of periprocedural MI had a 5-year mortality rate of 12.6%, compared with 8.4% in those without periprocedural MI, with an adjusted HR for mortality of 1.58.[2]

These data show that the association between MI and outcomes is present using both the Universal and SCAI definitions. The Universal definition seems to be more sensitive and identifies more patients with MI, whereas the SCAI definition identifies fewer patients. However, the MIs identified by the SCAI definition are larger in magnitude and associated with worse long-term outcomes.

MECHANISMS OF PERIPROCEDURAL MYOCARDIAL INFARCTION

The mechanisms of periprocedural MI include acute side branch occlusion, distal embolization resulting in slow flow or no reflow phenomenon, and abrupt vessel closure due to acute

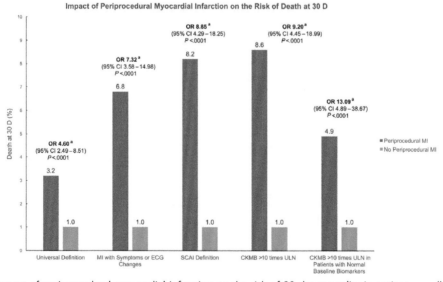

Fig. 1. Impact of periprocedural myocardial infarction on the risk of 30-day mortality in patients enrolled in the Cangrelor versus Standard Therapy to Achieve Optimal Management of Platelet Inhibition (CHAMPION PHOENIX) trial.[a] Adjusted for treatment, age, heart failure, diabetes, prior MI, country, and PCI duration. CI, confidence interval; CK-MB, creatine kinase-muscle/brain; ECG, electrocardiogram; MI, myocardial infarction; OR, odds ratio; PCI, percutaneous coronary intervention; SCAI, Society for Cardiovascular Angiography and Interventions; ULN, upper limit of normal. (Adapted from Cavender MA, Bhatt DL, Stone GW, et al. Consistent reduction in periprocedural myocardial infarction with cangrelor as assessed by multiple definitions: findings from CHAMPION PHOENIX (Cangrelor Versus Standard Therapy to Achieve Optimal Management of Platelet Inhibition). Circulation 2016;134(10):730; with permission.)

thrombosis of other mechanical processes such as dissection (Fig. 2).[11,40] Acute side branch occlusion is the most common mechanism of periprocedural MI.[11,40] Acute side branch occlusion can be caused by plaque shift from the parent vessel into the side branch, embolization from the parent vessel into the side branch, acute thrombosis in the side branch, dissection involving the side branch, and vasospasm involving the side branch during PCI of the parent vessel.[41–45] The origin of a side branch within the diseased segment of the parent vessel and the presence of a significant stenosis (>50%) within the ostium of a side branch are associated with an increased risk of acute side branch occlusion.[41–45] A side branch with a large diameter at baseline has a decreased risk of acute and chronic side branch occlusion.[43] The use of predilation, stent deployment with pressure inflation, high-pressure postdilation, the number of inflations, and the maximal inflation pressure are not associated with acute side branch occlusion.[43]

Distal embolization occurs frequently during PCI. Studies in which filter devices are placed distal to the target lesion have found that almost 3 out of 4 patients have some evidence of distal embolization.[46,47] The intentional plaque disruption, compression, fragmentation, and/or dissection at the target lesion from balloon angioplasty, atherectomy, or stent deployment can cause distal embolization of atheromatous and/or thrombotic debris, leading to microvascular obstruction, dysfunction, and ultimately MI.[46–53] Patients with acute coronary syndrome, evidence of thrombus, thin-cap fibroatheromas, and revascularization complicated by coronary artery dissection have higher rates of distal embolization and likelihood of periprocedural MI.[52,54] In addition to distal embolization, plaque disruption during PCI leads to a significant release of tissue factor and potent vasoconstrictors from macrophages and activated platelets.[55–58] Tissue factor activates the coagulation cascade with subsequent thrombin generation and also causes platelet activation and aggregation. This leads to further microvascular obstruction and dysfunction via the formation of microvascular thrombi. The released vasoconstrictors stimulate alpha-adrenergic receptors in the microcirculation, leading to neurohormonal activation and impairment of microvascular autoregulation with subsequent microvascular vasospasm.

Slow flow or no reflow phenomenon typically occurs immediately after balloon inflation or stent implantation and leads to angiographic evidence of contrast that slowly leaves or fails to leave in the coronary artery (TIMI 0 flow).[59,60] This is considered to be abrupt vessel closure when there is TIMI grade flow 0, with no angiographic evidence of contrast penetration past

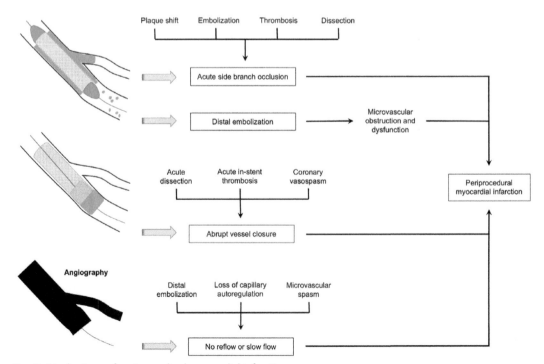

Fig. 2. Mechanisms of periprocedural myocardial infarction.

the target lesion, immediately after balloon angioplasty or stent implantation in a vessel in which flow had previously been present. It is caused most commonly by acute dissection and/or thrombosis and less commonly by coronary vasospasm.[61–63]

Plaque disruption from balloon angioplasty, atherectomy, or stent implantation can cause an acute dissection with subsequent intramural hemorrhage in the false lumen, leading to subsequent extrinsic compression against the true lumen and severe intracoronary flow limitation.[63] In severe circumstances, the dissection flap can cause an acute mechanical obstruction leading to the absence of distal intracoronary flow in the true lumen.[63] The intentional plaque disruption from PCI can also lead to acute thrombosis, especially in the setting of acute coronary syndromes, preexisting thrombus, severe residual stenosis, or ineffective periprocedural antithrombotic therapy.[63,64] Embolization of plaque and thrombus into the distal vessel and/or microvasculature, loss of capillary autoregulation, and microvascular spasm are all thought to be part of the pathophysiology of slow flow or no reflow.[60] TIMI grade flow 0 or 1 in the intervention vessel before PCI, increased plaque volume, increased change in plaque volume during stent implantation, and renal failure are all associated with an increased risk of no reflow.[59,60,65]

Although these are the most common causes of periprocedural MI, in some cases there is an asymptomatic increase in cardiac biomarkers without an identifiable cause.[11,40] In these circumstances, it is thought that the mechanism is most commonly distal embolization resulting in microvascular obstruction.

PREDICTORS OF PERIPROCEDURAL MYOCARDIAL INFARCTION

Predictors of periprocedural MI include factors related to the patient, lesion, and the procedure itself. Patients with advanced age, female gender, multivessel coronary artery disease (CAD), diffuse CAD, systemic atherosclerosis, diabetes mellitus, chronic and end-stage renal disease, and preprocedural cardiac biomarker elevation are at increased risk of periprocedural MI.[3,11,18,66–68] Anatomic factors associated with an increased risk of periprocedural MI include lesions of the left main and left anterior descending arteries, bifurcation lesions, calcified lesions, lesions longer than 20 mm, advanced CAD (high Syntax score), complex lesions (American College of Cardiology/American Heart Association [ACC/AHA] type C), lesions with high thrombus burden, and saphenous vein graft (SVG) lesions.[3,66,69] Multivessel interventions, bifurcation interventions, interventions of long lesions, and SVG interventions are also associated with an increased risk of periprocedural MI.[3,66,69]

PREVENTATIVE STRATEGIES

Strategies designed to reduce the risk of periprocedural MI focus on preventing intracoronary thrombus that forms from either a direct result of the intervention or through the formation of thrombus on equipment used to perform PCI. Antiplatelet therapies and anticoagulation significantly lower the risk of ischemic events in all patients undergoing PCI and are the cornerstone of pharmacologic therapies used in patients undergoing PCI (Fig. 3).[70] Devices designed to reduce thrombotic burden (eg, aspiration catheters) or to prevent distal embolization have not been shown to be effective when used routinely; however, some of these devices continue to have a role on a case-by-case basis.

Current antiplatelet therapies used in clinical practice include aspirin, oral $P2Y_{12}$ inhibitors (clopidogrel, prasugrel, ticagrelor), intravenous $P2Y_{12}$ inhibitors (cangrelor), and glycoprotein IIb/IIIa inhibitors (GPIs) (abciximab, eptifibatide, tirofiban). Aspirin, a cyclooxygenase-1 inhibitor, has been shown to reduce thrombus formation in patients undergoing PCI.[71] Current ACC/AHA guidelines recommend that all patients undergoing PCI who are not on daily aspirin should be given 325 mg before PCI.[72] The optimal dose following PCI remains a subject of debate. In the PCI-Clopidogrel in Unstable angina to prevent Recurrent Events (CURE) study, patients treated with 101 to 199 mg of aspirin or high dose ($\geq$200 mg) had similar rates of cardiovascular events when compared with patients treated with low-dose aspirin; however, bleeding was much higher in patients treated with low-dose aspirin.[73] Similar results were found in the Clopidogrel optimal loading dose Usage to Reduce Recurrent EveNTs-Organization to Assess Strategies in Ischemic Syndromes (CURRENT-OASIS-7) trial in which there was no difference in efficacy (or safety) with high (325 mg) versus low (75–100 mg daily) dose.[74] As a result, low-dose (<100 mg) aspirin is currently used indefinitely following PCI and is likely the adequate therapy for use in the periprocedural period for those patients who are on chronic aspirin therapy.

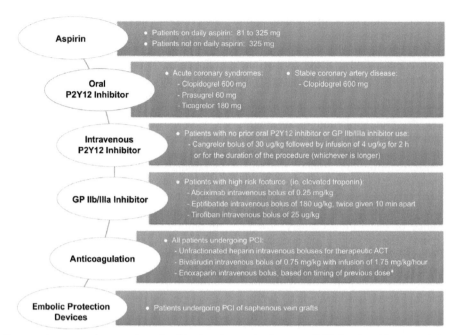

Fig. 3. Preventative strategies to reduce the risk of periprocedural myocardial infarction. ª Enoxaparin is given as a bolus of 0.5 to 0.75 mg/kg in patients who did not receive prior anticoagulation or a bolus of 0.3 mg/kg in those who received only one dose of enoxaparin before PCI or one dose of enoxaparin 8 to 12 hours before PCI; it is not given to those who received enoxaparin within 8 hours before PCI. GP, glycoprotein.

P2Y$_{12}$ inhibitors prevent platelet activation through the inhibition of adenosine diphosphate receptors and are also indicated in all patients undergoing PCI.[72,75] The utility of P2Y$_{12}$ inhibition in patients undergoing PCI was first seen with ticlopidine and has also been demonstrated with the P2Y$_{12}$ inhibitors that are currently available. For patients with stable coronary artery disease, clopidogrel is currently the recommended P2Y$_{12}$ inhibitor, whereas ticagrelor and prasugrel are preferred for patients with acute coronary syndrome. Whether patients undergoing PCI need pretreatment with P2Y$_{12}$ inhibitors remains an area of debate.[76,77] However, there is a clear relationship between increased platelet inhibition at the time of intervention and a decrease in the risk of ischemic events.[78,79]

In the subgroup of patients undergoing PCI in the CURE trial (n = 2658), pretreatment with clopidogrel reduced subsequent cardiovascular events. The benefits of clopidogrel were seen early, including less need for GPIs during PCI. Similar findings were found in the Clopidogrel for the Reduction of Events During Observation (CREDO) trial, which randomized patients undergoing PCI to either a clopidogrel loading dose (300 mg) or placebo. Patients who were treated with clopidogrel more than 6 hours before the PCI had lower rates of death, MI, or urgent target vessel revascularization at

28 days. The optimal dose of clopidogrel was explored in the Intracoronary Stenting and Antithrombotic Regimen: Choose between 3 High Oral Doses for Immediate Clopidogrel Effect (ISAR-CHOICE) trial, which found that 600 mg of clopidogrel had greater platelet inhibition when compared with 300 mg of clopidogrel and similar rates when compared with 900 mg.[80] The more potent P2Y$_{12}$ inhibitors, prasugrel and ticagrelor, have been found to reduce the risk of long-term risk of cardiovascular death, MI, or stroke in patients with acute coronary syndromes compared with clopidogrel but have not been well studied in stable ischemic heart disease.[81,82] Although the seminal trials with prasugrel and ticagrelor did include patients who were systematically pretreated before PCI, specific trials evaluating pretreatment with these agents did not observe reduction in major adverse cardiovascular events in patients undergoing PCI. In the Administration of Ticagrelor in the Cath Lab or in the Ambulance for New ST Elevation Myocardial Infarction to Open the Coronary Artery (ATLANTIC) study, although the rates of major adverse cardiovascular events did not differ significantly, patients who were pretreated with ticagrelor 180 mg loading dose had significantly lower rates of stent thrombosis compared with those who received ticagrelor 180 mg loading

dose in the cardiac catheterization laboratory at the time of PCI.[83]

The European Society of Cardiology (ESC) Guidelines on Myocardial Revascularization recommend clopidogrel 600 mg to be given in elective PCI patients once anatomy is known and the decision is made to proceed with PCI (preferably ≥2 hours or more before the PCI) (Class I Recommendation, Level of Evidence: A).[84] In patients with NSTE-ACS, guidelines recommend prasugrel (60 mg loading dose) in patients in whom coronary anatomy is known and who are proceeding to PCI or ticagrelor (180 mg loading dose) regardless of initial treatment strategy (invasive vs conservative), including those pretreated with clopidogrel (Class I Recommendation, Level of Evidence: B). The American College of Cardiology (ACC)/American Heart Association (AHA) guidelines state that a loading dose of a $P2Y^{12}$ receptor inhibitor should be given to patients undergoing PCI with stenting (Class I, Level of Evidence: A); however, recommendations regarding timing are not given.[72]

Cangrelor, an intravenous $P2Y_{12}$ inhibitor, has a rapid onset and offset of action and is approved for use in patients undergoing PCI who have not been pretreated with an oral $P2Y_{12}$ inhibitor. The CHAMPION PHOENIX trial included 11,145 patients who were undergoing PCI and had not been pretreated with a $P2Y_{12}$ inhibitor and randomized them to either cangrelor or clopidogrel. At 48 hours, patients treated with clopidogrel had lower rates of death, MI, ischemia-driven revascularization, or stent thrombosis (4.7% vs 5.9%, OR 0.78; 95% CI, 0.66–0.93; $P = .005$) with no difference in the risk of severe bleeding.[21,79] Similar results were found in a meta-analysis, which included all patients studied in the CHAMPION trials and found that cangrelor reduced the risk of death, MI, ischemia driven revascularization, or stent thrombosis (3.8% vs 4.7%; OR 0.81, 95% CI 0.71–0.91, $P = .0007$) and stent thrombosis (0.5% vs 0.8%, OR 0.59, 95% CI 0.43–0.80, $P = .0008$).[85] Cangrelor can be given as an intravenous weight-based bolus of 30 ug/kg followed by a weight-based infusion of 4 ug/kg for at least 2 hours or for the duration of the procedure, whichever is longer.[79]

Before the routine use of $P2Y_{12}$ inhibitors, intravenous GPIs were used as adjunctive antiplatelet therapy in patients undergoing PCI. GPIs inhibit platelet aggregation by interacting with the glycoprotein II/IIIa complex, either as an antibody (abciximab) or small molecule (tirofiban, eptifibatide), resulting in the inhibition of platelet cross-linking and subsequent aggregation.[86] Although some early studies found reductions in ischemic events, particularly in patients with elevated levels of cardiac troponin, more contemporary studies such as EARLY-ACS and ACUITY-TIMING found that the routine, upstream use of GPIs did not reduce ischemic events but did significantly increase the risk of bleeding.[87–91] Currently there are 3 GPIs available for use in clinical practice (abciximab, eptifibatide, and tirofiban). The most recent ESC guidelines do not recommend use of these agents on a routine basis, but support their use as bailout therapy in patients undergoing PCI in the case of intraprocedural thrombus, slow flow, or threatened vessel closure. Abciximab is given as an intravenous weight-based bolus of 0.25 mg/kg, eptifibatide as 2 intravenous weight-based boluses of 180 ug/kg 10 minutes apart, or tirofiban as an intravenous weigh-based bolus of 25 ug/kg.[72] Some studies have also found that intracoronary abciximab (0.25 mg/kg body weight) led to lower rates of surrogate endpoints and might be considered in patients with high thrombus burden.[92–95] Randomized studies to date evaluating the use of intracoronary fibrinolytics have not shown clinical benefit.[96]

Inhibitors of the coagulation cascade (unfractionated heparin–indirect thrombin inhibitor; enoxaparin–low-molecular-weight heparin; bivalirudin–direct thrombin inhibitor) are also given during PCI in order to reduce the risk of thrombotic complications.[70,72] Intravenous unfractionated heparin (UFH) is the predominant agent used in patients undergoing PCI.[97] Most of the data supporting the use of UFH are retrospective or from randomized trials when compared with other anticoagulants. When used as an adjunctive therapy in patients undergoing PCI, UFH is given as an intravenous weight-based bolus of 70 to 100 units/kg if no GPI is used or 50 to 70 units/kg if a GPI is used.[72] The activated clotting time (ACT) is checked periodically during PCI to monitor UFH's therapeutic effect because it is a mixture of polysaccharides with different molecular weights and can have variable bioavailability with different therapeutic responses between patients. One pooled analysis from randomized trials demonstrated the lowest ischemic event rates in patients with ACT values ranging from 350 to 375 seconds and the lowest bleeding event rates in patients with ACT values ranging from 300 to 350 seconds; another pooled analysis showed an increased bleeding risk with increasing ACT values and no significant association between ischemic events and ACT values.[98,99] During PCI, additional boluses of unfractionated heparin are given to achieve therapeutic levels if the ACT is less than 200 seconds in the setting of GPI use or 250 to 300 seconds in the absence of GPI use.[72]

Bivalirudin is a direct thrombin inhibitor that has been studied in patients undergoing PCI for stable angina, NSTE-ACS, and STEMI. Most of the trials evaluating bivalirudin have compared it to a regimen of heparin plus routine GPI. These studies largely found that bivalirudin was either noninferior or superior with regard to a composite primary endpoint of which included both ischemic and bleeding outcomes (death, MI, target-vessel revascularization for ischemia, stroke, or major bleeding); the main difference in outcomes between bivalirudin and UFH/GPI has been in the rates of bleeding events. In a large meta-analysis, a bivalirudin-based regimen increased the risk of periprocedural events including MI and stent thrombosis compared with a heparin-based regimen, but decreased the risk of bleeding. However, the differences in bleeding between bivalirudin and heparin regimens entirely depended on the proportion of patients treated with GPI in the heparin group.[100] Bivalirudin should be considered in patients who are at high risk of bleeding including those in whom GPI are planned, patients undergoing transfemoral access, or those in whom the procedural duration is expected to be long in order to minimize the need for ACT monitoring.[101] When used in patients undergoing PCI, it should be given as an intravenous weight-based bolus of 0.75 mg/kg followed by an intravenous weight-based infusion of 1.75 mg/kg per hour.[72]

Enoxaparin is another periprocedural anticoagulant that can be used in patients undergoing PCI. In the STEEPLE trial, 3528 patients undergoing PCI were randomized to receive enoxaparin (0.5 or 0.75 mg/kg of body weight) or unfractionated heparin. As compared with patients treated with heparin, 0.5 mg/kg of enoxaparin reduced the risk of bleeding at 48 hours with no difference in a composite endpoint of death or MI (HR 1.02; $P = .91$). ESC guidelines support its use as an anticoagulant in patients with stable angina (Class IIa, Level of Evidence: B), patients with NSTE-ACS who are already pretreated with enoxaparin (Class IIa, Level of Evidence: B) and in STEMI (Class IIb, Level of Evidence: B). The dosage of enoxaparin for ACS is 1 mg/kg given subcutaneously every 12 hours. In the United States, enoxaparin is not routinely used as adjunctive therapy for PCI because it is not easily possible to monitor the therapeutic coagulation with activated clotting times. In situations in which enoxaparin has been given for the treatment of ACS, it can be used as adjunctive therapy for PCI. It is administered as an intravenous weight-based bolus of 0.5 mg/kg in patients who have not received any prior anticoagulation or 0.3 mg/kg in those who received only one dose of subcutaneous enoxaparin before PCI or in those patients whose last dose of enoxaparin was 8 to 12 hours before PCI. Patients treated with more than one dose of subcutaneous enoxaparin and who received enoxaparin within 8 hours of the PCI do not need additional dosing.[72]

In addition to pharmacologic measures to reduce periprocedural MI, there are a variety of adjunctive devices that can also be used during the PCI procedure. Atherectomy with either orbital or rotational devices does not reduce the incidence of MI but may facilitate stent delivery and optimization. Thrombus aspiration, when used routinely in patients with MI, has not been shown to reduce events and may increase the risk of stroke; however, aspiration thrombectomy can be considered in patients with a heavy thrombus burden who are at high risk of distal embolization and no reflow. Embolic protection devices (EPDs) are designed to reduce plaque debris from reaching the microvascular circulation and causing periprocedural MI.[102] Several trials have shown that EPD use during SVG intervention reduces the risk of major adverse cardiac events and periprocedural MI; their use in SVG interventions is supported by ACC/AHA guidelines.[72,103–105]

SUMMARY

Periprocedural MI, irrespective of how defined or the magnitude of biomarker elevation, is associated with increased risk of morbidity and mortality. Understanding the mechanisms and predictors of periprocedural MI can help identify patients who would benefit from therapies that reduce the risk of ischemic events. Effective strategies to prevent periprocedural events include adequate platelet inhibition at the time of PCI with either early/upfront use of oral P2Y$_{12}$ inhibitors or intravenous cangrelor in those patients undergoing PCI who have not been pretreated with a P2Y$_{12}$ inhibitor and appropriately dosed intraprocedural anticoagulation.

REFERENCES

1. Benjamin EJ, Blaha MJ, Chiuve SE, et al. Heart disease and stroke statistics-2017 update: a report

from the American Heart Association. Circulation 2017;135(10):e146–603.

2. Cho MS, Ahn JM, Lee CH, et al. Differential rates and clinical significance of periprocedural myocardial infarction after stenting or bypass surgery for multivessel coronary disease according to various definitions. JACC Cardiovasc Interv 2017;10(15): 1498–507.

3. Zhang D, Li Y, Yin D, et al. Risk stratification of periprocedural myocardial infarction after percutaneous coronary intervention: analysis based on the SCAI definition. Catheter Cardiovasc Interv 2017;89(S1):S34–40.

4. Selvanayagam JB, Porto I, Channon K, et al. Troponin elevation after percutaneous coronary intervention directly represents the extent of irreversible myocardial injury: insights from cardiovascular magnetic resonance imaging. Circulation 2005;111(8):1027–32.

5. Andron M, Stables RH, Egred M, et al. Impact of periprocedural creatine kinase-MB isoenzyme release on long-term mortality in contemporary percutaneous coronary intervention. J Invasive Cardiol 2008;20(3):108–12.

6. Cavallini C, Savonitto S, Violini R, et al. Impact of the elevation of biochemical markers of myocardial damage on long-term mortality after percutaneous coronary intervention: results of the CK-MB and PCI study. Eur Heart J 2005;26(15):1494–8.

7. Ioannidis JP, Karvouni E, Katritsis DG. Mortality risk conferred by small elevations of creatine kinase-MB isoenzyme after percutaneous coronary intervention. J Am Coll Cardiol 2003;42(8): 1406–11.

8. Jang JS, Hong MK, Park DW, et al. Impact of periprocedural myonecrosis on clinical events after implantation of drug-eluting stents. Int J Cardiol 2008;129(3):368–72.

9. Jang JS, Jin HY, Seo JS, et al. Prognostic value of creatine kinase-myocardial band isoenzyme elevation following percutaneous coronary intervention: a meta-analysis. Catheter Cardiovasc Interv 2013;81(6):959–67.

10. Kini AS, Lee P, Marmur JD, et al. Correlation of postpercutaneous coronary intervention creatine kinase-MB and troponin I elevation in predicting mid-term mortality. Am J Cardiol 2004;93(1): 18–23.

11. Park DW, Kim YH, Yun SC, et al. Frequency, causes, predictors, and clinical significance of peri-procedural myocardial infarction following percutaneous coronary intervention. Eur Heart J 2013;34(22):1662–9.

12. Brener SJ, Ellis SG, Schneider J, et al. Frequency and long-term impact of myonecrosis after coronary stenting. Eur Heart J 2002; 23(11):869–76.

13. Lindsey JB, Kennedy KF, Stolker JM, et al. Prognostic implications of creatine kinase-MB elevation after percutaneous coronary intervention: results from the Evaluation of Drug-Eluting Stents and Ischemic Events (EVENT) registry. Circ Cardiovasc Interv 2011;4(5):474–80.

14. Feldman DN, Kim L, Rene AG, et al. Prognostic value of cardiac troponin-I or troponin-T elevation following nonemergent percutaneous coronary intervention: a meta-analysis. Catheter Cardiovasc Interv 2011;77(7):1020–30.

15. Feldman DN, Minutello RM, Bergman G, et al. Relation of troponin I levels following nonemergent percutaneous coronary intervention to short- and long-term outcomes. Am J Cardiol 2009; 104(9):1210–5.

16. Fuchs S, Kornowski R, Mehran R, et al. Prognostic value of cardiac troponin-I levels following catheter-based coronary interventions. Am J Cardiol 2000;85(9):1077–82.

17. Nienhuis MB, Ottervanger JP, Bilo HJ, et al. Prognostic value of troponin after elective percutaneous coronary intervention: a meta-analysis. Catheter Cardiovasc Interv 2008;71(3):318–24.

18. Prasad A, Rihal CS, Lennon RJ, et al. Significance of periprocedural myonecrosis on outcomes after percutaneous coronary intervention: an analysis of preintervention and postintervention troponin T levels in 5487 patients. Circ Cardiovasc Interv 2008;1(1):10–9.

19. Testa L, Van Gaal WJ, Biondi Zoccai GG, et al. Myocardial infarction after percutaneous coronary intervention: a meta-analysis of troponin elevation applying the new universal definition. QJM 2009; 102(6):369–78.

20. Tricoci P, Newby LK, Clare RM, et al. Prognostic and practical validation of current definitions of myocardial infarction associated with percutaneous coronary intervention. JACC Cardiovasc Interv 2018;11(9):856–64.

21. Cavender MA, Bhatt DL, Stone GW, et al. Consistent reduction in periprocedural myocardial infarction with cangrelor as assessed by multiple definitions: findings from CHAMPION PHOENIX (cangrelor versus standard therapy to achieve optimal management of platelet inhibition). Circulation 2016;134(10):723–33.

22. Group TS. The thrombolysis in myocardial infarction (TIMI) trial. Phase I findings. N Engl J Med 1985;312(14):932–6.

23. Mehta RH, Ou FS, Peterson ED, et al. Clinical significance of post-procedural TIMI flow in patients with cardiogenic shock undergoing primary percutaneous coronary intervention. JACC Cardiovasc Interv 2009;2(1):56–64.

24. Caixeta A, Lansky AJ, Mehran R, et al. Predictors of suboptimal TIMI flow after primary angioplasty

for acute myocardial infarction: results from the HORIZONS-AMI trial. EuroIntervention 2013;9(2): 220–7.

25. Gibson CM, Cannon CP, Murphy SA, et al. Relationship of TIMI myocardial perfusion grade to mortality after administration of thrombolytic drugs. Circulation 2000;101(2):125–30.

26. Henriques JP, Zijlstra F, van 't Hof AW, et al. Angiographic assessment of reperfusion in acute myocardial infarction by myocardial blush grade. Circulation 2003;107(16):2115–9.

27. Tricoci P. Consensus or controversy?: Evolution of criteria for myocardial infarction after percutaneous coronary intervention. Clin Chem 2017; 63(1):82–90.

28. Thygesen K, Alpert JS, Jaffe AS, et al. Fourth universal definition of myocardial infarction (2018). J Am Coll Cardiol 2018;72(18):2231–64.

29. Moussa ID, Klein LW, Shah B, et al. Consideration of a new definition of clinically relevant myocardial infarction after coronary revascularization: an expert consensus document from the Society for Cardiovascular Angiography and Interventions (SCAI). J Am Coll Cardiol 2013;62(17):1563–70.

30. Adams JE 3rd, Bodor GS, Davila-Roman VG, et al. Cardiac troponin I. A marker with high specificity for cardiac injury. Circulation 1993;88(1):101–6.

31. Goodman SG, Steg PG, Eagle KA, et al. The diagnostic and prognostic impact of the redefinition of acute myocardial infarction: lessons from the Global Registry of Acute Coronary Events (GRACE). Am Heart J 2006;151(3):654–60.

32. Lin JC, Apple FS, Murakami MM, et al. Rates of positive cardiac troponin I and creatine kinase MB mass among patients hospitalized for suspected acute coronary syndromes. Clin Chem 2004;50(2):333–8.

33. Jeremias A, Baim DS, Ho KK, et al. Differential mortality risk of postprocedural creatine kinase-MB elevation following successful versus unsuccessful stent procedures. J Am Coll Cardiol 2004;44(6):1210–4.

34. Bonaca MP, Wiviott SD, Braunwald E, et al. American College of Cardiology/American Heart Association/European Society of Cardiology/World Heart Federation universal definition of myocardial infarction classification system and the risk of cardiovascular death: observations from the TRITON-TIMI 38 trial (Trial to Assess Improvement in Therapeutic Outcomes by Optimizing Platelet Inhibition With Prasugrel-Thrombolysis in Myocardial Infarction 38). Circulation 2012;125(4):577–83.

35. Iakovou I, Mintz GS, Dangas G, et al. Increased CK-MB release is a "trade-off" for optimal stent implantation: an intravascular ultrasound study. J Am Coll Cardiol 2003;42(11):1900–5.

36. Prasad A, Gersh BJ, Bertrand ME, et al. Prognostic significance of periprocedural versus spontaneously occurring myocardial infarction after percutaneous coronary intervention in patients with acute coronary syndromes: an analysis from the ACUITY (Acute Catheterization and Urgent Intervention Triage Strategy) trial. J Am Coll Cardiol 2009;54(5):477–86.

37. Cavallini C, Verdecchia P, Savonitto S, et al. Prognostic value of isolated troponin I elevation after percutaneous coronary intervention. Circ Cardiovasc Interv 2010;3(5):431–5.

38. Miller WL, Garratt KN, Burritt MF, et al. Baseline troponin level: key to understanding the importance of post-PCI troponin elevations. Eur Heart J 2006;27(9):1061–9.

39. Tricoci P, Leonardi S, White J, et al. Cardiac troponin after percutaneous coronary intervention and 1-year mortality in non-ST-segment elevation acute coronary syndrome using systematic evaluation of biomarker trends. J Am Coll Cardiol 2013; 62(3):242–51.

40. Park DW, Kim YH, Yun SC, et al. Impact of the angiographic mechanisms underlying periprocedural myocardial infarction after drug-eluting stent implantation. Am J Cardiol 2014;113(7): 1105–10.

41. Arora RR, Raymond RE, Dimas AP, et al. Side branch occlusion during coronary angioplasty: incidence, angiographic characteristics, and outcome. Cathet Cardiovasc Diagn 1989;18(4): 210–2.

42. Meier B, Gruentzig AR, King SB 3rd, et al. Risk of side branch occlusion during coronary angioplasty. Am J Cardiol 1984;53(1):10–4.

43. Poerner TC, Kralev S, Voelker W, et al. Natural history of small and medium-sized side branches after coronary stent implantation. Am Heart J 2002; 143(4):627–35.

44. Vetrovec GW, Cowley MJ, Wolfgang TC, et al. Effects of percutaneous transluminal coronary angioplasty on lesion-associated branches. Am Heart J 1985;109(5 Pt 1):921–5.

45. Aliabadi D, Tilli FV, Bowers TR, et al. Incidence and angiographic predictors of side branch occlusion following high-pressure intracoronary stenting. Am J Cardiol 1997;80(8):994–7.

46. Angelini A, Rubartelli P, Mistrorigo F, et al. Distal protection with a filter device during coronary stenting in patients with stable and unstable angina. Circulation 2004;110(5):515–21.

47. Grube E, Gerckens U, Yeung AC, et al. Prevention of distal embolization during coronary angioplasty in saphenous vein grafts and native vessels using porous filter protection. Circulation 2001;104(20): 2436–41.

48. Ahmed JM, Mintz GS, Weissman NJ, et al. Mechanism of lumen enlargement during intracoronary stent implantation: an intravascular ultrasound study. Circulation 2000;102(1):7–10.

49. Bose D, von Birgelen C, Zhou XY, et al. Impact of atherosclerotic plaque composition on coronary microembolization during percutaneous coronary interventions. Basic Res Cardiol 2008;103(6): 587–97.

50. Kawamoto T, Okura H, Koyama Y, et al. The relationship between coronary plaque characteristics and small embolic particles during coronary stent implantation. J Am Coll Cardiol 2007;50(17):1635–40.

51. Dussaillant GR, Mintz GS, Pichard AD, et al. Effect of rotational atherectomy in noncalcified atherosclerotic plaque: a volumetric intravascular ultrasound study. J Am Coll Cardiol 1996;28(4):856–60.

52. Prati F, Pawlowski T, Gil R, et al. Stenting of culprit lesions in unstable angina leads to a marked reduction in plaque burden: a major role of plaque embolization? A serial intravascular ultrasound study. Circulation 2003;107(18):2320–5.

53. Saber RS, Edwards WD, Bailey KR, et al. Coronary embolization after balloon angioplasty or thrombolytic therapy: an autopsy study of 32 cases. J Am Coll Cardiol 1993;22(5):1283–8.

54. Porto I, Di Vito L, Burzotta F, et al. Predictors of periprocedural (type IVa) myocardial infarction, as assessed by frequency-domain optical coherence tomography. Circ Cardiovasc Interv 2012; 5(1):89–96. S1-6.

55. Gasperetti CM, Gonias SL, Gimple LW, et al. Platelet activation during coronary angioplasty in humans. Circulation 1993;88(6):2728–34.

56. Kereiakes DJ, Gurbel PA. Peri-procedural platelet function and platelet inhibition in percutaneous coronary intervention. JACC Cardiovasc Interv 2008;1(2):111–21.

57. Mahemuti A, Meneveau N, Seronde MF, et al. Early changes in local hemostasis activation following percutaneous coronary intervention in stable angina patients: a comparison between drug-eluting and bare metal stents. J Thromb Thrombolysis 2009;28(3):333–41.

58. Salloum J, Tharpe C, Vaughan D, et al. Release and elimination of soluble vasoactive factors during percutaneous coronary intervention of saphenous vein grafts: analysis using the PercuSurge GuardWire distal protection device. J Invasive Cardiol 2005;17(11):575–9.

59. Kotani J, Nanto S, Mintz GS, et al. Plaque gruel of atheromatous coronary lesion may contribute to the no-reflow phenomenon in patients with acute coronary syndrome. Circulation 2002;106(13): 1672–7.

60. Kelly RV, Cohen MG, Runge MS, et al. The no-reflow phenomenon in coronary arteries. J Thromb Haemost 2004;2(11):1903–7.

61. Detre KM, Holmes DR Jr, Holubkov R, et al. Incidence and consequences of periprocedural occlusion. The 1985-1986 National Heart, Lung, and Blood Institute Percutaneous Transluminal Coronary Angioplasty Registry. Circulation 1990;82(3): 739–50.

62. Lincoff AM, Popma JJ, Ellis SG, et al. Abrupt vessel closure complicating coronary angioplasty: clinical, angiographic and therapeutic profile. J Am Coll Cardiol 1992;19(5):926–35.

63. Bergelson BA, Fishman RF, Tommaso CL. Abrupt vessel closure: changing importance, management, and consequences. Am Heart J 1997; 134(3):362–81.

64. Bittl JA, Ahmed WH. Relation between abrupt vessel closure and the anticoagulant response to heparin or bivalirudin during coronary angioplasty. Am J Cardiol 1998;82(8B):50P–6P.

65. Katayama T, Kubo N, Takagi Y, et al. Relation of atherothrombosis burden and volume detected by intravascular ultrasound to angiographic no-reflow phenomenon during stent implantation in patients with acute myocardial infarction. Am J Cardiol 2006;97(3):301–4.

66. Kini A, Marmur JD, Kini S, et al. Creatine kinase-MB elevation after coronary intervention correlates with diffuse atherosclerosis, and low-to-medium level elevation has a benign clinical course: implications for early discharge after coronary intervention. J Am Coll Cardiol 1999;34(3): 663–71.

67. Batchelor WB, Anstrom KJ, Muhlbaier LH, et al. Contemporary outcome trends in the elderly undergoing percutaneous coronary interventions: results in 7,472 octogenarians. National Cardiovascular Network Collaboration. J Am Coll Cardiol 2000;36(3):723–30.

68. Marso SP, Gimple LW, Philbrick JT, et al. Effectiveness of percutaneous coronary interventions to prevent recurrent coronary events in patients on chronic hemodialysis. Am J Cardiol 1998;82(3): 378–80.

69. van Gaal WJ, Ponnuthurai FA, Selvanayagam J, et al. The syntax score predicts peri-procedural myocardial necrosis during percutaneous coronary intervention. Int J Cardiol 2009;135(1):60–5.

70. Rao SV, Ohman EM. Anticoagulant therapy for percutaneous coronary intervention. Circ Cardiovasc Interv 2010;3(1):80–8.

71. Barnathan ES, Schwartz JS, Taylor L, et al. Aspirin and dipyridamole in the prevention of acute coronary thrombosis complicating coronary angioplasty. Circulation 1987;76(1):125–34.

72. Levine GN, Bates ER, Blankenship JC, et al. 2011 ACCF/AHA/SCAI guideline for percutaneous coronary intervention. A report of the American College of Cardiology Foundation/American Heart Association Task Force on Practice Guidelines and the Society for Cardiovascular Angiography and Interventions. J Am Coll Cardiol 2011;58(24): e44–122.

73. Jolly SS, Pogue J, Haladyn K, et al. Effects of aspirin dose on ischaemic events and bleeding after percutaneous coronary intervention: insights from the PCI-CURE study. Eur Heart J 2009;30(8): 900–7.

74. Investigators C-O, Mehta SR, Bassand JP, et al. Dose comparisons of clopidogrel and aspirin in acute coronary syndromes. N Engl J Med 2010; 363(10):930–42.

75. Lilly SM, Wilensky RL. Emerging therapies for acute coronary syndromes. Front Pharmacol 2011;2:61.

76. Valgimigli M. Pretreatment with P2Y12 inhibitors in non-ST-segment-elevation acute coronary syndrome is clinically justified. Circulation 2014; 130(21):1891–903 [discussion: 1903].

77. Suda A, Namiuchi S, Kawaguchi T, et al. A simple and rapid method for identification of lesions at high risk for the no-reflow phenomenon immediately before elective coronary stent implantation. Heart Vessels 2016;31(12):1904–14.

78. Steinhubl SR, Berger PB, Brennan DM, et al. Optimal timing for the initiation of pre-treatment with 300 mg clopidogrel before percutaneous coronary intervention. J Am Coll Cardiol 2006; 47(5):939–43.

79. Bhatt DL, Stone GW, Mahaffey KW, et al. Effect of platelet inhibition with cangrelor during PCI on ischemic events. N Engl J Med 2013;368(14): 1303–13.

80. von Beckerath N, Taubert D, Pogatsa-Murray G, et al. Absorption, metabolization, and antiplatelet effects of 300-, 600-, and 900-mg loading doses of clopidogrel: results of the ISAR-CHOICE (intracoronary stenting and antithrombotic regimen: choose between 3 high oral doses for immediate clopidogrel effect) trial. Circulation 2005;112(19): 2946–50.

81. Wiviott SD, Braunwald E, McCabe CH, et al. Prasugrel versus clopidogrel in patients with acute coronary syndromes. N Engl J Med 2007;357(20): 2001–15.

82. Wallentin L, Becker RC, Budaj A, et al. Ticagrelor versus clopidogrel in patients with acute coronary syndromes. N Engl J Med 2009;361(11):1045–57.

83. Montalescot G, van 't Hof AW, Lapostolle F, et al. Prehospital ticagrelor in ST-segment elevation myocardial infarction. N Engl J Med 2014; 371(11):1016–27.

84. Authors/Task Force Members, Windecker S, Kolh P, Alfonso F, et al. 2014 ESC/EACTS guidelines on myocardial revascularization: The Task Force on Myocardial Revascularization of the European Society of Cardiology (ESC) and the European Association for Cardio-Thoracic Surgery (EACTS)Developed with the special contribution of the European Association of Percutaneous Cardiovascular Interventions (EAPCI). Eur Heart J 2014;35(37):2541–619.

85. Steg PG, Bhatt DL, Hamm CW, et al. Effect of cangrelor on periprocedural outcomes in percutaneous coronary interventions: a pooled analysis of patient-level data. Lancet 2013;382(9909): 1981–92.

86. Chew DP, Moliterno DJ. A critical appraisal of platelet glycoprotein IIb/IIIa inhibition. J Am Coll Cardiol 2000;36(7):2028–35.

87. Kastrati A, Mehilli J, Neumann FJ, et al. Abciximab in patients with acute coronary syndromes undergoing percutaneous coronary intervention after clopidogrel pretreatment: the ISAR-REACT 2 randomized trial. JAMA 2006;295(13): 1531–8.

88. Tcheng JE, Kandzari DE, Grines CL, et al. Benefits and risks of abciximab use in primary angioplasty for acute myocardial infarction: the Controlled Abciximab and Device Investigation to Lower Late Angioplasty Complications (CADILLAC) trial. Circulation 2003;108(11):1316–23.

89. Topol EJ, Byzova TV, Plow EF. Platelet GPIIb-IIIa blockers. Lancet 1999;353(9148):227–31.

90. Giugliano RP, White JA, Bode C, et al. Early versus delayed, provisional eptifibatide in acute coronary syndromes. N Engl J Med 2009;360(21):2176–90.

91. Stone GW, Bertrand ME, Moses JW, et al. Routine upstream initiation vs deferred selective use of glycoprotein IIb/IIIa inhibitors in acute coronary syndromes: the ACUITY Timing trial. JAMA 2007; 297(6):591–602.

92. Mehilli J, Kastrati A, Schulz S, et al. Abciximab in patients with acute ST-segment-elevation myocardial infarction undergoing primary percutaneous coronary intervention after clopidogrel loading: a randomized double-blind trial. Circulation 2009;119(14):1933–40.

93. Wohrle J, Grebe OC, Nusser T, et al. Reduction of major adverse cardiac events with intracoronary compared with intravenous bolus application of abciximab in patients with acute myocardial infarction or unstable angina undergoing coronary angioplasty. Circulation 2003;107(14):1840–3.

94. Deibele AJ, Jennings LK, Tcheng JE, et al. Intracoronary eptifibatide bolus administration during percutaneous coronary revascularization for acute coronary syndromes with evaluation of platelet glycoprotein IIb/IIIa receptor occupancy and

platelet function: the Intracoronary Eptifibatide (ICE) Trial. Circulation 2010;121(6):784–91.

95. Stone GW, Maehara A, Witzenbichler B, et al. Intracoronary abciximab and aspiration thrombectomy in patients with large anterior myocardial infarction: the INFUSE-AMI randomized trial. JAMA 2012;307(17):1817–26.

96. Morales-Ponce FJ, Lozano-Cid FJ, Martinez-Romero P, et al. Intracoronary Tenecteplase versus Abciximab as adjunctive treatment during primary percutaneous coronary intervention in patients with anterior myocardial infarction. EuroIntervention 2018. [Epub ahead of print].

97. Zeymer U, Rao SV, Montalescot G. Anticoagulation in coronary intervention. Eur Heart J 2016; 37(45):3376–85.

98. Chew DP, Bhatt DL, Lincoff AM, et al. Defining the optimal activated clotting time during percutaneous coronary intervention: aggregate results from 6 randomized, controlled trials. Circulation 2001;103(7):961–6.

99. Brener SJ, Moliterno DJ, Lincoff AM, et al. Relationship between activated clotting time and ischemic or hemorrhagic complications: analysis of 4 recent randomized clinical trials of percutaneous coronary intervention. Circulation 2004; 110(8):994–8.

100. Cavender MA, Sabatine MS. Bivalirudin versus heparin in patients planned for percutaneous coronary intervention: a meta-analysis of randomised controlled trials. Lancet 2014;384(9943): 599–606.

101. Cavender MA, Faxon DP. Can BRIGHT restore the glow of bivalirudin? JAMA 2015;313(13):1323–4.

102. Bangalore S, Bhatt DL. Embolic protection devices. Circulation 2014;129(17):e470–6.

103. Baim DS, Wahr D, George B, et al. Randomized trial of a distal embolic protection device during percutaneous intervention of saphenous vein aorto-coronary bypass grafts. Circulation 2002; 105(11):1285–90.

104. Mauri L, Cox D, Hermiller J, et al. The PROXIMAL trial: proximal protection during saphenous vein graft intervention using the Proxis Embolic Protection System: a randomized, prospective, multicenter clinical trial. J Am Coll Cardiol 2007; 50(15):1442–9.

105. Stone GW, Rogers C, Hermiller J, et al. Randomized comparison of distal protection with a filter-based catheter and a balloon occlusion and aspiration system during percutaneous intervention of diseased saphenous vein aorto-coronary bypass grafts. Circulation 2003;108(5): 548–53.

Culprit-Only or Complete Revascularization for ST-Elevation Myocardial Infarction in Patients with and Without Shock

Mark K. Tuttle, MD, Duane S. Pinto, MD, MPH*

KEYWORDS

- Nonculprit percutaneous coronary intervention • STEMI • Complete revascularization
- Cardiogenic shock

KEY POINTS

- ST-elevation myocardial infarction (STEMI) patients with multivessel disease and without shock are a common clinical entity, but the best approach to nonculprit vessel lesions remains controversial.
- STEMI patients with shock do not appear to benefit from primary multivessel percutaneous coronary interventions (PCIs) during the index procedure.
- The optimal treatment strategy in a given STEMI patient involves an individualized approach, incorporating clinical, hemodynamic, and angiographic/imaging parameters.
- Patients with STEMI and cardiogenic shock may benefit from therapies other than PCI, such as mechanical cardiovascular support.

INTRODUCTION

Cardiogenic shock complicates an increasing number of ST-elevation myocardial infarctions (STEMIs),[1] but despite advances in management strategies, the mortality in affected patients approaches 50%.[2] Management decisions are particularly important early in the course of illness, given that, of all STEMI patients treated with percutaneous coronary intervention (PCI), 76% of deaths within the first week are due to cardiogenic shock.[3] Because multivessel coronary artery disease (CAD) is present in 40% to 65% of all STEMI patients[4,5] and up to 80% of patients with STEMI complicated by cardiogenic shock,[6] the decision regarding whether to perform PCI in diseased, non-infarct-related arteries (non-IRAs) in addition to the culprit vessel is a common clinical dilemma. The purpose of this review is to summarize clinical trial data to aid the clinician in determining the optimal revascularization strategy for STEMI patients with multivessel disease.

DEFINITIONS AND TERMINOLOGY

A detailed discussion of culprit-only or complete revascularization in the setting of STEMI requires familiarity with a set of definitions and terminology (Box 1).

PATHOPHYSIOLOGY

Cellular and Physiologic Processes

The pathologic processes in STEMI result in a self-perpetuating decline in cardiac performance.

Disclosure Statement: Dr D.S. Pinto serves as a consultant for Medtronic and Boston Scientific.
Beth Israel Deaconess Medical Center, Harvard Medical School, 185 Pilgrim Road, West Campus, Baker 4, Boston, MA 02215, USA
* Corresponding author.
E-mail address: dpinto@bidmc.harvard.edu

2211-7458/19/© 2019 Elsevier Inc. All rights reserved.

> **Box 1**
> **Common definitions and terminology**
>
> - Culprit lesion: Angiographic coronary stenosis or occlusion corresponding to the suspected ischemic territory and thus thought to explain the acute clinical presentation during acute myocardial infarction (MI).
> - Infarct-related artery (IRA): Coronary artery containing the culprit lesion.
> - Non-infarct-related artery (non-IRA): Vessels comprising the remainder of the coronary tree that do not contain the culprit lesion.
> - Complete revascularization: Relieving all coronary stenoses of a given severity (variably defined).
>   - Multivessel primary percutaneous coronary intervention (MV PPCI): Performing complete revascularization during the index PCI procedure.
>   - Staged PCI: Performing PCI of diseased non-IRA vessels at a time other than the index PCI procedure.

Because ischemia results in tissue hypoxia and thus impaired cellular production of adenosine triphosphate, there is systolic and diastolic myocardial dysfunction leading to increased left ventricular end diastolic pressure (LVEDP). This process decreases coronary perfusion pressure (CPP) (CPP = diastolic blood pressure − LVEDP)[7] and increases myocardial oxygen consumption,[8] which in turn leads to further ischemia. Concurrently, myocardial necrosis leads to release of inflammatory mediators, such as interleukin-6, which impairs contractility and reduces catecholamine responsiveness.[9]

Macroscopic Processes

An extensive territory of affected myocardium is often required to result in cardiogenic shock. Acute myocardial infarction (MI) patients with shock had a greater amount of affected left ventricular mass (51%) compared with those without shock (23%)[10]; as expected, those with shock and extensive infarcts more frequently had 3-vessel CAD (54%) than those without shock (20%).[10] Extensive infarction results in reduced contractile function, diastolic dysfunction, and decreased cardiac output with associated malperfusion.

Separately, valvular dysfunction may occur in the form of annular dilation or tethered/restricted leaflet motion depending on the location and size of the infarct. In the case of an infarcted papillary muscle, frank rupture and flail leaflet mitral regurgitation may result. Finally, as a later complication, myocardial wall rupture or ventricular septal rupture can occur, frequently with a catastrophic outcome. It is unlikely that nonculprit PCI improves or avoids mechanical complications of MI, but it is postulated that non-IRA PCI would improve left ventricular contractile performance if the myocardium supplied by the non-IRA is ischemic.

THE DILEMMA

Particularly in those cases with cardiogenic shock involving large ischemic territories, it stands to reason that restoring normal blood flow to all coronary arteries with flow-limiting lesions would provide maximal benefit. The potential benefits of complete revascularization include minimizing the infarct size, preserving ventricular function, reducing ischemia-related arrhythmias, and preventing future ischemic events.

However, the theoretic advantages of complete revascularization have not been uniformly observed in all subsets of patients. Lack of observed benefit may be due to the potential drawbacks of multivessel PCI, which include greater contrast use (and thus nephropathy), increased risk of stent thrombosis, and longer procedure time as well as a lack of benefit in repairing arteries that are not flow limiting (Table 1).

ST-ELEVATION MYOCARDIAL INFARCTION WITHOUT CARDIOGENIC SHOCK
Synopsis of Current Data

There have been 4 contemporary randomized trials of PCI strategies in patients with STEMI and multivessel CAD in the absence of cardiogenic shock (Table 2). All were relatively small

> **Table 1**
> **Theoretic benefits of culprit-only versus complete revascularization in ST-elevation myocardial infarction**

Culprit-Only Revascularization	Complete Revascularization
- Reduced contrast use	- Minimize infarct size
- Reduced risk of stent thrombosis	- Preserve ventricular function
- Reduced risk of procedural complications	- Arrhythmia reduction
- Shorter procedure time	- Prevent recurrent ischemia/infarction

Randomized trials of percutaneous coronary intervention strategies in ST-elevation myocardial infarction patients with multivessel disease without shock

	Politi et al,[17] 2010	PRAMI (2013)[18]	CvLPRIT (2015)[20]	DANAMI-3 PRIMULTI (2015)[21]
Inclusion criteria	• STEMI ≤12 h • Multivessel CAD (>70% stenosis in ≥2 coronary arteries)	• STEMI or new left bundle branch block • Successful PCI • Multivessel CAD with ≥50% stenosis in ≥1 other artery suitable for PCI	• STEMI ≤12 h • Referred for PPCI • Multivessel CAD with >1 vessel >2 mm in diameter with >70% stenosis in 1 plane or >50% stenosis in 2 planes • Non-IRA suitable for stent implantation	• STEMI ≤12 h • Successful IRA PPCI • >50% stenosis >2 mm in non-IRA suitable for PCI
Exclusion criteria	• Cardiogenic shock • LMCA disease ≥50% • Prior CABG • Severe valvular disease • Unsuccessful PPCI	• Cardiogenic shock • LMCA equivalent disease (LM or ostial LAD and LCx >50% stenosis) • Prior CABG • Non-IRA CTO	• Indication/contraindication to complete revascularization • Prior Q-wave MI • Prior CABG • Shock, VSD, ≥ moderate MR • Chronic kidney disease • Stent thrombosis • CTO of the only non-IRA	• Cardiogenic shock • Hemodynamic instability or ischemia in non-IRA territory • CTO of non-IRA
Number of participants	N = 214	N = 465	N = 296	N = 627
Shock patients	Excluded	Excluded	Excluded	Excluded
Intervention(s)	• PPCI followed by staged PCI of diseased non-IRAs • MV PPCI	• MV PCI in non-IRA with >50% stenosis at the time of PPCI	• MV PCI either at time of PPCI (72% of patients) or as a staged in-hospital procedure (28% of patients)	• Complete in-hospital revascularization with staged MV PCI for lesions >90% and staged FFR-guided MV PCI for lesions 50%–90% stenosis
Comparator	Culprit-only revascularization	Culprit-only revascularization	Culprit-only revascularization	Culprit-only revascularization
Outcome measure	MACE at 2.5 y (cardiac or noncardiac death, in-hospital death, reinfarction, rehospitalization for ACS, repeat coronary revascularization)	MACE at 23 mo (death, MI, refractory angina)	Composite of death, recurrent MI, CHF, and ischemia-driven revascularization at 12 mo	MACE at 12 mo (death, MI, ischemia-driven revascularization of non-RA lesions)
Findings	• Primary endpoint: 23.1% with CR vs 20% with SR vs 50% in the COR (P<.001) • All-cause mortality: 9.2% with CR vs 6.2% with SR vs 15.5% with COR (P = NS)	• Primary endpoint: 9% with MV PCI vs 23% with COR (P<.001) • All-cause mortality: 5.1% with MV PCI vs 6.9% with R (P = NS)	• Primary endpoint: 10% with MV PCI vs 21.2% with COR (P = .009) • 12-mo mortality: 2.7% with MV PCI vs 6.9% with COR (P = .09)	• Primary endpoint: 13% with MV PCI vs 22% with COR (P = .004) • 12-mo mortality: 5% with MV PCI vs 4% with COR (P = .43)

Abbreviations: CR, complete revascularization; COR, culprit-only revascularization; LAD, left anterior descending; LBBB, left bundle branch block; LCx, left circumflex; LM, left main; LMCA, left main coronary artery; NS, not significant; SR, staged revascularization; VSD, ventricular septal defect.

(between 214 and 627 participants). Each demonstrated a statistically significant benefit of complete revascularization over culprit-only revascularization in terms of major adverse cardiovascular events (MACE) (defined differently in each trial), and none showed a reduction in all-cause mortality. There was heterogeneity in the specifics of patient selection, the timing of revascularization of diseased non-IRAs (MV PPCI, staged non-IRA PCI, or a hybrid approach), and the definitions of clinical endpoints, although the general approach in each trial was similar.

Rationale for Treatment of Non-Infarct-Related Arteries

The apparent benefit of treating non-IRA lesions, as demonstrated by these 4 trials, differs from the results of the COURAGE trial,[11] which suggested that PCI may not prevent death or MI in stable CAD. One theory for this discrepancy is that the degree of remote ischemia may be greater in diseased non-IRA territories during the stress of STEMI compared with similar lesions in stable patients. Furthermore, the benefit of revascularizing arteries that subtend large ischemic territories is evidenced by a substudy of COURAGE, which showed that the benefit of PCI was greater among patients with the most ischemia on perfusion imaging.[12]

Another theory offered to distinguish the role of revascularization in stable CAD versus acute coronary syndrome (ACS) relates to inflammation. Proponents of this theory argue that ACS is a decidedly distinct pathophysiologic process, involving widespread inflammation of the coronary tree,[13] which may result in the rare occurrence of multiple plaque rupture events (2.5% in one series[14]). As such, the benefit of performing PCI of seemingly bystander non-IRA lesions in STEMI would be to prevent plaque rupture during this vulnerable time period of acute inflammation. Intravascular imaging assessment of plaque morphology in ACS patients supports this theory. In a study comparing optical coherence tomography characteristics of nonculprit plaques in patients with ACS versus stable angina, investigators demonstrated that fibrous cap was significantly thinner in nonculprit lesions in ACS patients than in stable angina patients.[15] In the PROSPECT (Providing Regional Observations to Study Predictors of Events in the Coronary Tree: An Imaging Study in Patients With Unstable Atherosclerotic Lesions) study of 697 ACS patients who underwent 3-vessel imaging with intravascular ultrasonography, subsequent MACE events attributed to non-IRAs were not infrequent in long-term follow-up; subsequent MACE events were adjudicated to be related to culprit lesions in 12.9% of patients and to nonculprit lesions in 11.6% at 3 years.[16]

Summary of Randomized Trials

Politi and colleagues[17] conducted a randomized trial of 214 patients with STEMI and multivessel CAD. Patients were randomized to one of 3 strategies: MV PPCI, PPCI followed by staged PCI of diseased non-IRAs, or culprit-only revascularization. The primary endpoint, a composite of mortality, in-hospital death, reinfarction, rehospitalization for ACS, or repeat coronary revascularization, was observed more frequently in the culprit-only revascularization arm (50%) compared with the staged PCI arm (20%) and the MV PPCI arm (23.1%). All-cause mortality was no different among the study arms. The rate of contrast-induced nephropathy was also similar across groups in this population with mostly normal renal function.

The Randomized Trial of Preventive Angioplasty (PRAMI) study[18] randomized 465 patients with STEMI and multivessel CAD to MV PPCI or culprit-only PCI. At a median follow-up of 23 months, the primary endpoint of a composite of death, MI, or refractory angina was seen in 9% of patients with MV PCI versus 23% of patients with culprit-only revascularization ($P<.001$). When examined individually, both cardiovascular death (1.7% vs 4.3%, $P = .07$) and nonfatal MI (3% vs 8.7%, $P = .009$) were lower in the MV PPCI group. Although procedure time, radiation dose, and contrast volume were higher in the MV PPCI arm compared with the culprit-only revascularization arm, there was no difference in the rates of contrast nephropathy requiring dialysis (0.4% vs 1.3%, $P = .37$), procedure-related stroke (0.9% vs 0%, $P = .5$), or bleeding requiring transfusion or surgery (2.9% vs 2.6%, $P = .8$). The trial was stopped early by the Data and Safety Monitoring Committee because of the difference detected in the primary outcome, but critics speculate that had enrollment continued, the initial observed benefit may have narrowed. The study was terminated after 74 events had occurred (14 cardiac deaths, 27 nonfatal MIs, and 42 episodes of refractory angina [patients could be double-counted if they experienced multiple events]). Three more nonfatal MIs in the control arm would have resulted in a nonsignificant P value.[19] Other criticisms include the lack of description of lesion characteristics and the absence of a core laboratory angiographic analysis.

The Complete vs Lesion-Only Primary PCI Trial (CvLPRIT)[20] study randomized 296 patients with STEMI and multivessel CAD to complete revascularization (either MV PPCI or PPCI followed by staged non-IRA PCI) or culprit-only revascularization. The composite endpoint of death, recurrent MI, congestive heart failure (CHF), ischemia-driven revascularization occurred in 10% of the MV PCI group compared with 21.2% of patients in the culprit-only revascularization arm (P = .009.) There was no significant difference in mortality. As with PRAMI, in CvLPRIT, the complete revascularization arm had higher contrast volume and procedure duration but showed no difference in the safety endpoints of procedure-related stroke, major bleeding, or contrast nephropathy. Unfortunately, because the timing of non-IRA PCI was not specified in the study protocol, the optimal timing of non-IRA PCI (during the index procedure or staged procedure) remained unsettled.

The Third DANish Study of Optimal Acute Treatment of Patients with ST-segment Elevation Myocardial Infarction: PRImary PCI in MULTIvessel Disease (DANAMI-3 PRIMULTI)[21] trial randomized 627 patients with STEMI and multivessel CAD to complete revascularization (PPCI for lesions >90% and staged fractional flow reserve [FFR]-guided PCI for lesions 50% to 90%) or culprit-only revascularization. The incorporation of FFR stemmed from the idea that using physiologic guidance would limit PCI just to vessels that would otherwise have been at high risk of requiring urgent revascularization at a later date. Patients were followed for an average of 12 months for the primary composite endpoint of death, MI, ischemia-driven revascularization of non-IRA lesions. The primary endpoint occurred in 13% of those in the complete revascularization arm versus 22% in the culprit-only revascularization arm (P = .004). Critics argue that the use of FFR soon after MI may be unreliable due to altered microvascular resistance and reduced coronary flow reserve.[22] The FFR STABILITY study examined this concept by comparing the FFR values of non-IRAs during STEMI and during a subsequent catheterization (41.8 ± 10.2 days later) and found that mean FFR values decrease in follow-up, albeit by a small amount (0.84 ± 0.08 at initial presentation vs 0.82 ± 0.08 in follow-up, P = .025).[23] The implication is that FFR during ACS may result in false-negative results. As such, the benefit from revascularization of non-IRAs in DANAMI-3 PRIMULTI[21] may have been attenuated, and if there had been more reliable measurement of flow-limitation of non-IRAs during the index

ACS event, the treatment effect for non-IRA PCI may have been magnified.

ST-ELEVATION MYOCARDIAL INFARCTION WITH CARDIOGENIC SHOCK
Synopsis of Current Data
Two randomized trials of PCI strategies in STEMI complicated by cardiogenic shock have been conducted (Table 3). In contrast to that demonstrated by the trials of nonshock STEMI patients, a strategy of multivessel PCI in patients with shock appears to be harmful. The mechanism of this difference remains unknown. Some speculate that an increased incidence of no-reflow is to blame; because no-reflow occurs in up to 30% of STEMI cases,[24] this may be even more pronounced in cases of reduced global coronary blood flow, such as cardiogenic shock. Others suggest that because shock patients are frequently prescribed intravenous catecholamine therapies, which increase platelet reactivity, there may be an increased risk of stent thrombosis,[25] a risk that could be multiplicative when additional stents are deployed.

Summary of Randomized Trials
The Should We Emergently Revascularize Occluded Coronaries for Cardiogenic Shock (SHOCK trial)[26] included 302 STEMI patients with cardiogenic shock. Patients were randomized to early revascularization (thrombolysis, balloon angioplasty, stenting, or coronary artery bypass grafting [CABG]) within 6 hours or a medical stabilization strategy of thrombolytics and then possible revascularization 54 hours or more after randomization. Patients undergoing revascularization could undergo multivessel PCI or culprit-only revascularization at the discretion of the operator.[27] At 30 days, there was no difference in mortality between groups, but a mortality difference emerged at 6 months (50% with early revascularization vs 63.1% with delayed possible revascularization) and persisted in long-term follow-up.[28] This trial did not evaluate complete versus culprit-only revascularization in a systemic fashion.

The Culprit Lesion Only PCI vs Multivessel PCI in Cardiogenic Shock (CULPRIT-SHOCK trial)[6] randomized 686 STEMI patients with acute MI (STEMI or non-STEMI) to multivessel PPCI versus culprit-only PCI followed by the option of staged non-IRA PCI. Mortality was 43.3% in the culprit-only PPCI group compared with 51.6% in the MV PPCI group (P = .03); however, at 1-year follow-up, there was no difference in mortality between the 2 groups.[29] Critics of this study argue that

	SHOCK (1999)[26,27]	**CULPRIT-SHOCK (2017)**[6]
Table 3 Randomized trials of percutaneous coronary intervention strategies in ST-elevation myocardial infarction patients with multivessel disease and shock		
Inclusion criteria	• STEMI or new left bundle branch block • Systolic blood pressure (SBP)<90 mm Hg • End-organ hypoperfusion • CI <2.2 • PCWP ≥15 mm Hg	• STEMI or non-STEMI • Multivessel CAD with >1 vessel >2 mm in diameter with >70% stenosis with an identifiable culprit lesion • SBP <90 mm Hg for >30 min or the use of catecholamine therapy • Clinical signs of pulmonary congestion • End-organ hypoperfusion (altered mental status, cool extremities, oliguria, or lactate >2 mmol/L)
Exclusion criteria	• Severe systemic illness • Mechanical or other cause of shock • Isolated right ventricular failure • Severe valvular disease • Known dilated cardiomyopathy • Recent hemorrhage • Not a candidate for revascularization • Inability to obtain vascular access	• Resuscitation >30 min • No intrinsic heart action • Assumed severe deficit in cerebral function with fixed dilated pupils • Indication for primary CABG • A mechanical cause of shock • Onset of shock >12 h before randomization • Age >90 y • Massive pulmonary embolism • Severe renal failure (CCl<30 mL/min) • Other disease associated with survival <6 mo
Number of participants	N = 302	N = 686
Shock patients	Included	Included
Intervention	Early revascularization (thrombolysis, balloon angioplasty, or stenting) (culprit-only for 1 or 2-vessel disease, and operator discretion for 3-vessel disease) ≤6 h after randomization	Multivessel PCI at the time of PPCI
Comparator	Possible revascularization ≥54 h after randomization	Primary PCI of the culprit lesion only with the option of staged revascularization of nonculprit lesions
Outcome measures	• 30-d mortality • 6-mo mortality	• All-cause mortality or severe renal failure requiring RRT • All-cause mortality • Renal replacement therapy
Findings	• 30-d mortality: 46.7% with early revascularization vs 56% with possible delayed revascularization (P = .11) • 6-mo mortality: 50.3% with early revascularization vs 63.1% with delayed revascularization (P = .027) • Long-term follow-up (6 y) mortality[28]: 19.6% with early revascularization vs 32.8% with possible delayed revascularization	• Composite endpoint: 55.4% with MV PCI vs 45.9% with COR (P = .01) • All-cause mortality: 51.6% with MV PCI vs 43.3% with COR (P = .03) • Renal replacement therapy: MV PCI 16.4% vs 11.6% (P = .07)

Abbreviations: CI, cardiac index; CCl, creatinine clearance; PCWP, pulmonary capillary wedge pressure; RV, right ventricle; SBP, systolic blood pressure.

because chronic total occlusions (CTOs) were included and mandated to be attempted to be revascularized in the MV PPCI group, this may have conferred harm because the benefit of revascularization of CTOs in the setting of shock is unclear and the procedural risk is greater. Nevertheless, this study forms the basis of the updated 2018 European Society of Cardiology (ESC)/European Association for Cardio-Thoracic Surgery (EACTS) practice guidelines, dictating that routine revascularization of non-IRA lesions is not recommended during primary PCI (*Class II, Level of Evidence: B*) (Table 4).

APPROACH TO PERCUTANEOUS CORONARY INTERVENTION IN ST-ELEVATION MYOCARDIAL INFARCTION PATIENTS WITH MULTIVESSEL CORONARY ARTERY DISEASE

The optimal management strategy for STEMI patients with multivessel CAD involves incorporating knowledge of pathophysiology, clinical trial data, and common sense. As with any undertaking in medicine, this involves critical appraisal of the available data and developing an individualized strategy for a given patient. Possible PCI strategies include culprit-only revascularization or complete revascularization, with either culprit and non-IRA PCI during index procedure or culprit vessel PCI followed by staged PCI of non-IRA.

APPROACH TO THE ST-ELEVATION MYOCARDIAL INFARCTION PATIENT WITHOUT CARDIOGENIC SHOCK

Despite 4 randomized trials with supportive outcomes, the heterogeneity in their inclusion criteria and outcome measures limits the ability to arrive at a unifying approach that can be generalized to all patients. The largest, and most recent of these trials, DANAMI-3 PRIMULTI[21] seems to provide the most rational approach, perhaps because its design may have been informed by the pitfalls and criticisms of the prior 3 trials. The protocol for this trial mandated that only non-IRA lesions greater than 90% be intervened upon during the index PCI procedure in addition to the culprit lesion. This was followed by staged, FFR-guided PCI for lesions of 50% to 90% stenosis. This approach seems to balance the benefit of restoring flow in ischemic myocardium in the regions with the most flow-limiting stenosis while not expending excess fluoroscopy time, contrast volume, and catheter manipulation in intermediate 50% to 90% lesions that may or may not be truly flow limiting.

Quantitative angiographic studies suggest that non-IRAs can have worse-appearing stenoses during acute MI compared with follow-up angiography. This phenomenon may be related to transient vasoconstriction related to high circulating levels of catacholamines.[30] As such, decisions on revascularization of intermediate non-IRA lesions on the index procedure may be safely deferred to subsequent angiography and evaluation, thereby avoiding the oculostenotic reflex.[31] The operator must be able to balance the complexity of intervention with the anticipated benefit in a given patient at both the index and the subsequent procedures. For example, one must integrate a variety of factors beyond the severity of the stenosis and the presence of flow limitation, including the risk of repair (eg, chronic occlusion, calcification requiring atherectomy), the size of the territory involved, and the patient's associated comorbidities when making the decision of whether to perform PCI of non-IRA (Table 5).

APPROACH TO THE ST-ELEVATION MYOCARDIAL INFARCTION PATIENT WITH CARDIOGENIC SHOCK

Compared with other STEMI patients, those with cardiogenic shock have a greater burden of CAD, higher degree of organ dysfunction, and a substantially increased risk of mortality. Unlike their nonshock counterparts, in STEMI patients with shock, there is no benefit to upfront complete revascularization, and there may even be short-term harm with this strategy.[6] On the basis of CULPRIT-SHOCK,[6] and its long-term follow-up,[29] the ESC/EACTS have updated their practice guidelines to recommend against routine MV PPCI.

Table 4 Summary of practice guidelines for percutaneous coronary intervention of non-infarct-related arteries in ST-elevation myocardial infarction with shock	
ACCF/AHA Guidelines (2013)[34]	**ESC/EACTS Guidelines (2018)[33]**
• No specific recommendation is made about non-IRA revascularization in patients with shock	• In cardiogenic shock, routine revascularization of non-IRA lesions is not recommended during primary PCI (Class II, Level of Evidence: B)

Table 5
Summary of practice guidelines for percutaneous coronary intervention of non-infarct-related arteries in ST-elevation myocardial infarction without shock

American College of Cardiology/American Heart Association/Society for Cardiovascular Angiography and Interventions (AHA/ACC/SCAI) Guidelines Focused Update (2015)[32]	ESC/EACTS Guidelines (2018)[33]
• PCI of a noninfarct artery may be considered in selected patients with STEMI and multivessel disease who are hemodynamically stable, either at the time of primary PCI or as a planned staged procedure (Class IIb, Level of Evidence B-R)	• Routine revascularization of non-IRA lesions should be considered in STEMI patients with multivessel disease before hospital discharge. (Class IIa, Level of Evidence: A)

American College of Cardiology Foundation (ACCF)/AHA Guidelines (2013)[34]	
• PCI is indicated in a noninfarct artery at a time separate from primary PCI in patients who have spontaneous symptoms of ischemia (Class I, Level of Evidence C) • PCI is reasonable in a noninfarct artery at a time separate from primary PCI in patients with intermediate- or high-risk findings on noninvasive testing (Class IIa, Level of Evidence B)	

SURGICAL COMPLETE REVASCULARIZATION IN ST-ELEVATION MYOCARDIAL INFARCTION

Although the focus of this review has been PCI strategy, the authors note that CABG is also a strategy for complete revascularization. There are no randomized trials or large observational studies comparing PCI to CABG in STEMI. However, CABG has a limited role in the management of patients with STEMI given that fibrinolysis and/or primary PCI can restore coronary flow more rapidly than the time it takes to perform a CABG; in a modern cohort of STEMI patients, only 1.2% underwent CABG within 24 hours of STEMI, and just 5.5% underwent CABG within 30 days of STEMI[35] (Table 6).

FUTURE DIRECTIONS

The COMPLETE (Complete vs Culprit-only Revascularization to Treat Multivessel Disease After Primary PCI for STEMI) trial (ClinicalTrials.gov; #NCT01740479) will compare staged complete revascularization to culprit-only revascularization in 3900 STEMI patients. Given the significantly higher number of participants than prior trials, this study will be better powered to investigate hard endpoints such as mortality.

Regarding STEMI patients with cardiogenic shock, the decision of whether to revascularize a non-IRA is likely to be less important than other therapies offered. The authors theorize that aggressive resuscitative measures and management, which may involve invasive

Table 6
Summary of practice guidelines for coronary artery bypass grafting in ST-elevation myocardial infarction

AHA/ACC Guidelines (2013)[34]	ESC/EACTS Guidelines (2018)[33]
• Urgent CABG is indicated in patients with STEMI and coronary anatomy not amenable to PCI who have ongoing or recurrent ischemia, cardiogenic shock, severe HF, or other high-risk features (Class I, Level of Evidence: B) • CABG is recommended in patients with STEMI at time of operative repair of mechanical defects (Class I, Level of Evidence: B) • Emergency CABG within 6 h of symptom onset may be considered in patients with STEMI who do not have cardiogenic shock and are not candidates for PCI or fibrinolytic therapy. (Class IIb, Level of Evidence: C)	• CABG should be considered in patients with ongoing ischemia and large areas of jeopardized myocardium if PCI of the IRA cannot be performed. (Class IIa, Level of Evidence: C)

hemodynamic monitoring and mechanical support, may serve to improve outcomes where non-IRA PCI has not. A recent pilot study from the National Cardiogenic Shock Initiative, a protocolized, collaborative management strategy of patients with acute MI and cardiogenic shock, emphasizing early and liberal use of percutaneous ventricular assist device support before revascularization, has shown impressive results, with survival increasing from around 50% to 76%.[1] Although this is only observational data at present, it may represent a paradigm shift away from the ingrained emphasis on door-to-balloon time of revascularization and toward early left ventricular unloading and provision of mechanical circulatory support before PCI with close attention to management before and after the PCI procedure.

REFERENCES

1. Basir MB, Schreiber T, Dixon S, et al. Feasibility of early mechanical circulatory support in acute myocardial infarction complicated by cardiogenic shock: The Detroit cardiogenic shock initiative. Catheter Cardiovasc Interv 2018;91(3):454–61.

2. Nguyen HL, Yarzebski J, Lessard D, et al. Ten-year (2001-2011) trends in the incidence rates and short-term outcomes of early versus late onset cardiogenic shock after hospitalization for acute myocardial infarction. J Am Heart Assoc 2017;6(6). https://doi.org/10.1161/JAHA.117.005566.

3. Doost Hosseiny A, Moloi S, Chandrasekhar J, et al. Mortality pattern and cause of death in a long-term follow-up of patients with STEMI treated with primary PCI. Open Heart 2016;3(1):e000405.

4. Jaski BE, Cohen JD, Trausch J, et al. Outcome of urgent percutaneous transluminal coronary angioplasty in acute myocardial infarction: comparison of single-vessel versus multivessel coronary artery disease. Am Heart J 1992;124(6):1427–33.

5. Muller DW, Topol EJ, Ellis SG, et al. Thrombolysis and Angioplasty in Myocardial Infarction (TAMI) Study Group. Multivessel coronary artery disease: a key predictor of short-term prognosis after reperfusion therapy for acute myocardial infarction. Am Heart J 1991;121(4 Pt 1):1042–9.

6. Thiele H, Akin I, Sandri M, et al. PCI strategies in patients with acute myocardial infarction and cardiogenic shock. N Engl J Med 2017;377(25):2419–32.

7. Buchanan KD, Kolm P, Iantorno M, et al. Coronary perfusion pressure and left ventricular hemodynamics as predictors of cardiovascular collapse following percutaneous coronary intervention. Cardiovasc Revasc Med 2018. https://doi.org/10.1016/j.carrev.2018.09.005.

8. Baller D, Wolpers HG, Hoeft A, et al. Increase of myocardial oxygen consumption due to active diastolic wall tension. Basic Res Cardiol 1984;79(2):176–85.

9. Westaby S, Kharbanda R, Banning AP. Cardiogenic shock in ACS. Part 1: prediction, presentation and medical therapy. Nat Rev Cardiol 2011;9(3):158–71.

10. Alonso DR, Scheidt S, Post M, et al. Pathophysiology of cardiogenic shock. Quantification of myocardial necrosis, clinical, pathologic and electrocardiographic correlations. Circulation 1973;48(3):588–96.

11. Boden WE, O'Rourke RA, Teo KK, et al. Optimal medical therapy with or without PCI for stable coronary disease. N Engl J Med 2007;356(15):1503–16.

12. Shaw LJ, Berman DS, Maron DJ, et al. Optimal medical therapy with or without percutaneous coronary intervention to reduce ischemic burden: results from the Clinical Outcomes Utilizing Revascularization and Aggressive Drug Evaluation (COURAGE) trial nuclear substudy. Circulation 2008;117(10):1283–91.

13. Buffon A, Biasucci LM, Liuzzo G, et al. Widespread coronary inflammation in unstable angina. N Engl J Med 2002;347(1):5–12.

14. Pollak PM, Parikh SV, Kizilgul M, et al. Multiple culprit arteries in patients with ST segment elevation myocardial infarction referred for primary percutaneous coronary intervention. Am J Cardiol 2009;104(5):619–23.

15. Maejima N, Hibi K, Saka K, et al. Morphological features of non-culprit plaques on optical coherence tomography and integrated backscatter intravascular ultrasound in patients with acute coronary syndromes. Eur Heart J Cardiovasc Imaging 2015;16(2):190–7.

16. Stone GW, Maehara A, Lansky AJ, et al. A prospective natural-history study of coronary atherosclerosis. N Engl J Med 2011;364(3):226–35.

17. Politi L, Sgura F, Rossi R, et al. A randomised trial of target-vessel versus multi-vessel revascularisation in ST-elevation myocardial infarction: major adverse cardiac events during long-term follow-up. Heart 2010;96(9):662–7.

18. Wald DS, Morris JK, Wald NJ, et al. Randomized trial of preventive angioplasty in myocardial infarction. N Engl J Med 2013;369(12):1115–23.

19. Montori V. MSc. Scrutinizing the PRAMI Trial of "Preventive Angioplasty" - CardioExchange. CardioExchange. 2013. Available at: https://blogs.jwatch.org/cardioexchange/2013/09/26/scrutinizing-the-prami-trial-of-preventive-angioplasty/. Accessed October 9, 2018.

20. Gershlick AH, Khan JN, Kelly DJ, et al. Randomized trial of complete versus lesion-only revascularization in patients undergoing primary percutaneous coronary intervention for STEMI and multivessel

disease: the CvLPRIT trial. J Am Coll Cardiol 2015; 65(10):963–72.

21. Engstrøm T, Kelbæk H, Helqvist S, et al. Complete revascularisation versus treatment of the culprit lesion only in patients with ST-segment elevation myocardial infarction and multivessel disease (DANAMI-3—PRIMULTI): an open-label, randomised controlled trial. Lancet 2015;386(9994): 665–71.

22. Niccoli G, Indolfi C, Davies JE. Evaluation of intermediate coronary stenoses in acute coronary syndromes using pressure guidewire. Open Heart 2017;4(2):e000431.

23. Wood DA, Poulter R, Boone R, et al. Stability of non culprit vessel fractional flow reserve in patients with St-segment elevation myocardial infarction. Can J Cardiol 2013;29(10):S291–2.

24. Harrison RW, Aggarwal A, Ou F-S, et al. Incidence and outcomes of no-reflow phenomenon during percutaneous coronary intervention among patients with acute myocardial infarction. Am J Cardiol 2013;111(2):178–84.

25. Hochman JS, Katz S. Back to the future in cardiogenic shock - initial PCI of the culprit lesion only. N Engl J Med 2017;377(25):2486–8.

26. Hochman JS, Sleeper LA, Webb JG, et al. Early revascularization in acute myocardial infarction complicated by cardiogenic shock. SHOCK Investigators. Should we emergently revascularize occluded coronaries for cardiogenic shock. N Engl J Med 1999;341(9):625–34.

27. Hochman JS, Sleeper LA, Godfrey E, et al. SHould we emergently revascularize Occluded Coronaries for cardiogenic shocK: an international randomized trial of emergency PTCA/CABG-trial design. The SHOCK Trial Study Group. Am Heart J 1999; 137(2):313–21.

28. Hochman JS, Sleeper LA, Webb JG, et al. Early revascularization and long-term survival in cardiogenic shock complicating acute myocardial infarction. JAMA 2006;295(21):2511–5.

29. Thiele H, Akin I, Sandri M, et al. One-year outcomes after PCI strategies in cardiogenic shock. N Engl J Med 2018. https://doi.org/10.1056/NEJMoa1808788.

30. Hanratty CG, Koyama Y, Rasmussen HH, et al. Exaggeration of nonculprit stenosis severity during acute myocardial infarction: implications for immediate multivessel revascularization. J Am Coll Cardiol 2002;40(5):911–6.

31. Topol EJ. Coronary angioplasty for acute myocardial infarction. Ann Intern Med 1988;109(12):970.

32. Levine GN, Bates ER, Blankenship JC, et al. 2015 ACC/AHA/SCAI focused update on primary percutaneous coronary intervention for patients with ST-elevation myocardial infarction: an update of the 2011 ACCF/AHA/SCAI guideline for percutaneous coronary intervention and the 2013 ACCF/AHA guideline for the management of ST-elevation myocardial infarction. J Am Coll Cardiol 2016; 67(10):1235–50.

33. Neumann F-J, Sousa-Uva M, Ahlsson A, et al. 2018 ESC/EACTS Guidelines on myocardial revascularization. Eur Heart J 2018. https://doi.org/10.1093/eurheartj/ehy394.

34. Writing Committee Members, O'gara PT, Kushner FG, Ascheim DD, et al. 2013 ACCF/AHA guideline for the management of St-elevation myocardial infarction: a report of the American College of Cardiology Foundation/American Heart Association Task Force on Practice Guidelines. Circulation 2013. Available at: https://www.ahajournals.org/doi/abs/10.1161/CIR.0b013e3182742cf6. Accessed October 7, 2018.

35. Gu YL, van der Horst ICC, Douglas YL, et al. Role of coronary artery bypass grafting during the acute and subacute phase of ST-elevation myocardial infarction. Neth Heart J 2010;18(7–8):348–54.

Moving?

Make sure your subscription moves with you!

To notify us of your new address, find your **Clinics Account Number** (located on your mailing label above your name), and contact customer service at:

Email: journalscustomerservice-usa@elsevier.com

800-654-2452 (subscribers in the U.S. & Canada)
314-447-8871 (subscribers outside of the U.S. & Canada)

Fax number: 314-447-8029

Elsevier Health Sciences Division
Subscription Customer Service
3251 Riverport Lane
Maryland Heights, MO 63043

*To ensure uninterrupted delivery of your subscription, please notify us at least 4 weeks in advance of move.

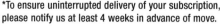

Printed and bound by CPI Group (UK) Ltd, Croydon, CR0 4YY

03/10/2024

01040307-0012